Caring for Arab Patients

Caring for Arab Patients
A BIOPSYCHOSOCIAL APPROACH

Edited by

LAETH SARI NASIR MBBS
Professor of Family Medicine, Department of Family Medicine
University of Nebraska Medical Center, Omaha, NE

and

ARWA KAYED ABDUL-HAQ MBBS, MSc (Peds), MFT
Staff Physician, Children's Hospital, Omaha, NE
Volunteer Faculty, Departments of Family Medicine and Pediatrics
University of Nebraska Medical Center, Omaha, NE

Foreword by

ALA TOUKAN MB, BS (Lond), FRCP(C)
Clinical Professor of Medicine and Gastroenterology
Former Dean, Faculty of Medicine
University of Jordan, Amman

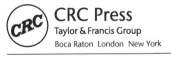

CRC Press
Taylor & Francis Group
Boca Raton London New York

CRC Press is an imprint of the
Taylor & Francis Group, an **informa** business

CRC Press
Taylor & Francis Group
6000 Broken Sound Parkway NW, Suite 300
Boca Raton, FL 33487-2742

© 2008 by Laeth S Nasir and Arwa K Abdul-Haq
CRC Press is an imprint of Taylor & Francis Group, an Informa business

First issued in paperback 2019

No claim to original U.S. Government works

ISBN 13: 978-0-367-44614-7 (pbk)
ISBN 13: 978-1-84619-182-4 (hbk)

Visit the Taylor & Francis Web site at
http://www.taylorandfrancis.com

and the CRC Press Web site at
http://www.crcpress.com

Contents

Part 3: Mental health

Part 4: Patient education

Foreword

Today medical practice in the Arab world is predominantly grounded in that of the Western model. Many healthcare providers have trained in Euro-American schools, and consequently the health infrastructure in the Arab world has been molded along similar lines. Graduating students and specialists from these Arab institutions are products of this model in their own countries.

On the other hand, the background culture and the inherent psychosocial dimension of the medical encounter remain poorly integrated factors in the health provision process. Thus the practice language is often foreign to the provider–patient exchange in the Arab world, while signs and symptoms are interpreted according to set definitions in Western textbooks. Many other familiar instances of this deficiency come to mind as examples. For instance, is the extended family's often overwhelming presence alongside the patient understood and used to advantage? Or is it seen as a troublesome manifestation in keeping with the Western concept of limiting such a role? How does the patient (and family) comprehend illness in terms of presentation to the healthcare provider and compliance with treatment? In this regard, "late presentation" and "poor compliance" are dismissals commonly expressed by the health provider with little thought given to the psychosocial appraisal of such failures. Analysis of these common scenarios may challenge and advance comprehension of the cultural milieu of healthcare, as well as teaching and research in the Arab world.

A call to highlight the cultural and psychosocial dimensions of medical practice in the Arab world should lead to a process of reorientation in this direction, preferably based on data from local studies rather than a process of learning by trial and error. To this end the authors of this book, experts on psychosocial impact of disease from Arab and Western institutions, have presented a remarkable effort in accumulating and analysing a surprising volume of studies done on this subject but which have not been collated for this purpose previously. They tackle many aspects in the dimension of cultural influences on medical practice, including issues where psychosocial factors are of primary importance in the disease setting (mental health issues), and others where these factors are a backdrop to the issue under care (culture, environment and health, the family).

Arab health providers are likely to read this book with an interest stimulated by familiarity with the issues, while simultaneously recognizing their own lack of comprehension of the subject. It is to be hoped that, in the near future, a critical mass of these health providers will call for the inclusion of this subject matter in curricula at all levels of education for those providing care to the citizens of the Arab world – the ultimate beneficiaries of a sound scientific and culturally relevant basis of health provision.

Ala Toukan MB, BS (Lond), FRCP(C)
Clinical Professor of Medicine and Gastroenterology
Former Dean, Faculty of Medicine
University of Jordan, Amman
January 2008

Preface

Caring for Arab Patients: a biopsychosocial approach is designed for physicians, medical students and other health professionals who work with patients in the Arab world.

The first text of its kind, *Caring for Arab Patients* uses a cross-disciplinary synthesis of research evidence to explore the psychosocial aspects of medical care in Arab countries. The contributors, who include distinguished scientists and academics from the region, provide fresh and authoritative analysis, clinical approaches and directions for further research. This book will be indispensable to those wishing to gain an understanding of the psychosocial dimensions of medical care in Arab countries.

Laeth S Nasir and Arwa K Abdul-Haq
January 2008

About the editors

Laeth S Nasir MBBS is a Professor of Family Medicine at the University of Nebraska Medical Center. A former Fulbright scholar, he has taught, studied and carried out research in the United States and the Arab world for over 20 years, and has written extensively on various topics in primary care.

Arwa K Abdul-Haq MBBS, MSc (Peds), MFT serves as volunteer faculty at the University of Nebraska Medical Center, and is a Staff Physician at the Children's Hospital in Omaha, Nebraska. A pediatrician and medical family therapist, she has special expertise in behavioral, developmental and learning problems in children, particularly within the context of their families. She has studied and researched the family in both the United States and the Arab world. She is currently working on a curriculum to integrate brief therapy models into primary care pediatric practice.

List of contributors

Dr Abdelrazzak Abyad MD, PhD, MPH, MBA, AGSF
Consultant in Family Medicine and Geriatrics
Editor, *Middle-East Journal of Family Medicine*
Editor, *Middle-East Journal of Age & Aging*
Editor, *Middle-East Journal of Business*
Chairman, Middle-East Academy for Medicine of Aging
Coordinator, Middle-East Primary Care Research Network
Coordinator, Middle-East Network on Ageing Research
President, Middle-East Association on Aging and Alzheimer's
Director, Abyad Medical Center and Middle East Longevity Institute
Tripoli-Lebanon

Dr Raeda Al-Qutob MBBS, MPH, DrPH
Professor and Associate Dean of Research and Development
University of Jordan, Amman

Dr Taysir Diab
Psychiatrist and Senior Researcher
Gaza Community Mental Health Program (GCMHP)
Gaza City

Dr Eyad El-Sarraj
Psychiatrist and General Director
Gaza Community Mental Health Program (GCMHP)
Gaza City

Dr Adib Essali MD, PhD, MRCPsych
Director
Center of Psychiatry
Damascus, Syria

Dr Aisha Hamdan PhD
Assistant Professor
College of Medicine
University of Sharjah
United Arab Emirates

Dr Sherine F Hamdy PhD
Department of Anthropology
Brown University
Providence, RI

Dr Brigitte Khoury PhD
Assistant Professor and Clinical Psychologist
Department of Psychiatry
American University of Beirut Medical Center

Dr Michel R Khoury MD, MA
American University of Beirut

Dr Anahid Kulwicki RN, DNS, FAAN
Professor
Wayne County Health and Human Services
Oakland University School of Nursing
Detroit, MI

Dr Nasser Shuriquie MD, MRCPsych
King Hussein Medical Center
Amman, Jordan

Dr Ghazi O Tadmouri PhD
Assistant Director
Centre for Arab Genomic Studies
Dubai, United Arab Emirates.

Dr Abdel Aziz Thabet
Psychiatrist and Senior Researcher
Gaza Community Mental Health Program (GCMHP)
Gaza City

Introduction

As we move into the 21st century, new health challenges are emerging that threaten to overwhelm the health systems of many developing countries. Issues that include aging populations, increases in the prevalence of chronic diseases, and social dysfunctions, are only a few of the problems that are emerging or projected to materialize as major health issues for Arab countries within the next few decades.

Psychosocial dimensions of medical care exert major impacts on health and treatment outcomes. While clinical approaches to most illnesses are easily transferable across cultures, many aspects of medical practice need modifications to fit different cultural settings. Understanding these problems and their solutions in the context of our own culture is important; uncritically employing Western models, paradigms and research to deal with many of these issues may result in outcomes that are not sustainable or well suited to our needs.

Our purpose in developing this text is twofold. The first is to explore scientific literature related to psychosocial aspects of medicine. There is a growing body of academic literature from disciplines such as sociology, psychology, anthropology and medicine addressing psychosocial factors that affect the medical encounter in the Arab world. This information has not been collected or synthesized in a form that can readily inform the education and practice of physicians and other healthcare professionals. Gathering this evidence to create a cross-disciplinary synthesis applicable to clinical practice will help to identify gaps and controversies in the literature, and may provide a framework for future research.

The second purpose of this book is to help to begin the process of systematically exploring and developing explanatory models of psychosocial determinants of health in our region. Exploring these issues with an appreciation of the adaptive functions that the existing dynamics represent for the individual, family and society will help us to develop approaches that more closely match the needs of people in our region. These new approaches, by taking advantage of the strengths inherent in our society, will help physicians and other health providers to enhance their ability to provide quality medical care to the patients and populations that they serve.

In developing this text, we have been fortunate to have received valuable support and input from exceptional academics and researchers from throughout the Arab world. With their help, we attempted to focus on issues that were felt to be most important in the clinical setting, or that had the potential to exert a disproportionate impact on the health of individuals, families and communities. We hope that future editions of this book will expand the breadth and scope of the topics presented here, and that new research and ideas will continue to enrich the delivery of medical care in our region.

PART 1

Culture, environment and health

CHAPTER 1

Culture and health

(★ *Sherine F Hamdy and Laeth S Nasir*

How can the study of "culture" help us to deliver better healthcare? Culture is defined as people's beliefs, customs, practices and social behavior. All aspects of life are affected by people's unique cultural perspectives, including their views of health, illness and medical treatment. Cultures are not just bounded units such as "the Arabs" or "the Chinese" or "Navajo Indians". Rather, specific sites within a society, such as "the medical profession", can foster their own culture which then affects the interactions between healthcare providers and their patients. There are many cultures in the Arab world. What we define as "culture" is a dynamic and fluid process, as people adapt to changes in their environment such as urbanization, education and mobility. Sometimes, rapid environmental changes outpace the capacity of cultures to adjust. This can create incompatibility between people and their environment, or can aggravate differences between generations within the same population.

Understanding the culture (of patients, healthcare providers, and the medical system itself) is crucial to delivering quality medical care. While signs of physical disease may be similar in different parts of the world, almost everything else in the medical encounter is different in different cultures. The meaning of illness, understanding of disease processes and health, treatment seeking behavior, compliance with medical treatment, and illness attribution all are culturally specific. The expression of psychological distress, its causes and effects on individuals and families is particularly related to cultural norms and values. Understanding the role of the family in the individual's health and welfare differs significantly between cultures and has considerable impact on the delivery of healthcare. Furthermore, the cultural understanding of the physician's role requires changes in the ways that medical advice and treatment are delivered and received.

Medical practices from Euro-American contexts may not always translate well into other societies, such as those in Arab countries. Governments invest money into the biomedical system of healthcare, with the presumption that new medical interventions and practices will be passively accepted by the recipients of this care. Yet often, they are subject to challenge and change by local perceptions, traditions and expectations. For example, the introduction of ultrasound into prenatal care in the public health system in an Arab country unexpectedly resulted in a greatly increased demand for prenatal services. Subsequently, it was discovered that many women and families were using ultrasound to discover the baby's sex antenatally. This resulted in unforeseen health outcomes[1] and required modifications in practice.

Culture is important because it affects the way we create, receive, process and interpret information. It influences how we perceive and express discomfort and suffering. By defining social structure and behavioral patterns, culture may affect the incidence and manifestations of certain diseases. Frequently culture shapes what does and does not qualify as "illness" in a given community. There are some cultural attitudes that negatively impact overall health. For example, some families insist that their children eat, as a sign of love. This is a continuation of cultural traditions that originated in environments of nutritional scarcity, when parents would sacrifice their portions to their children. Yet in a new environment, among middle-class urban families where abundant, highly caloric food is available, this same practice of "love" may lead to child obesity and to future health problems. This problem is exacerbated as work conditions outside the home and consumerism and advertising lead to the consumption of more pre-packaged and processed foods and to less active lifestyles. In some communities, women are discouraged from going outside the home regularly; in small urban spaces this confinement and alienation can lead to depression, anxiety, lack of exercise and obesity.

There are also cultural practices that positively affect health. For example, close family social support helps to prevent and alleviate many physical and psychological pressures. Many people's religious practices and beliefs give them a sense of security and strong sense of self. Arab countries are one of the few areas of the world where the prevalence of HIV and other sexually transmitted diseases is very low, due largely to strong social imperatives surrounding marriage and sexuality.

In a sociological study of medical doctors in Egypt, it was found that physicians cited "culture" as the number-one reason impeding the proper delivery of healthcare.[2] Often, they meant that villagers or lower-class patients were ignorant and that this ignorance prevented proper healthcare delivery and treatment. However, what is referred to as "ignorance" frequently reflects unrecognized incompatibility between the health provider's own medical and personal values and those of the patient. When viewed in this light, study of the social life, habits and beliefs of patients and communities becomes nearly as important as studying the biological features of disease. When providers understand their patients' values, social surroundings and living conditions, they can often provide better treatment and outcomes. Unfortunately, very little work on this aspect of medicine has been done in the Arab world; not infrequently, studies that have been done are flawed by the use of Western cultural explanatory models of motivation and behavior. For example, some authors report that traditional Western group psychotherapy may be harmful among some Arab patients.[3]

The following are some case studies to elucidate some ways in which social and cultural issues impact clinical practice.

Case study I: Elderly eye patient

Amina, an older peasant woman with cataracts, comes into the public eye hospital because she cannot see well and she requests eye drops. When she hears the word "surgery" from the doctor, she refuses adamantly. She says that only God is the Healer, and that she is too old for these things. The attending doctor says it is "hopeless" with older rural women because of their "ignorance" and moves on to the next patient.

Analysis

Amina is reacting negatively to the word "surgery" because, in her experience, there have not been good medical resources and people have not had good surgical outcomes. She has heard many stories of people suffering from post-surgical complications and poor medical treatment. She does not want to become an inpatient in a hospital where she may be poorly treated by the nurses and staff. She is afraid of anesthesia at her age, and does not want to die in a hospital. The doctors seem indifferent to her concerns. Furthermore, she cannot afford to spend any resources on herself – any extra money that she has she prefers to spend on her children and their families.

It is clear that, in this case, it is not "ignorance" preventing the woman from seeking treatment but previous negative experiences with medical treatment. Past negative experiences with medical treatments resonate powerfully in close-knit communities. People know each other well and the suffering of one member of the community may be quickly communicated, and acutely felt by others. One first-hand story of success or failure may likely be much more powerful in shaping perceptions about the risk of a procedure than statistical data. The doctor might reassure Amina and her family that improved health would benefit not only herself but also her family members and community. By eliciting unspoken concerns and modifying the way relevant information is communicated, the physician can help this patient and her family to assess honestly the risks and benefits in her case.

Importantly, the problem of Amina points to much larger structural problems that cannot be adequately addressed in a physician–patient encounter. For those committed to improving healthcare in the Arab world, there needs to be large-scale commitment to the provision of better healthcare institutions, better funding and resources, and better social services for poor patients.

Case study II: Young woman in obstetrics

Samira comes to the hospital requesting obstetric treatment. She tells the doctor that she is suffering from infertility and that she wants a laparascopic examination done. Upon interview, the doctor learns that this patient has been married for only six weeks.

Analysis

There is strong cultural pressure on Samira, and on many others, to become pregnant immediately after marriage. The neighbors and her in-laws have already begun talking about her and making her feel bad that she has not yet become pregnant. The patient should receive counseling to help her understand that there is nothing wrong with her or her body. Although infertility may be attributed to either male or female factors, it is often women who are assumed socially to be the "problem". Samira and her husband could be counseled together and given social support. It is important to communicate with this patient because she has stated that she will seek treatment at private clinics to get faster results. Some physicians in these private clinics perform unnecessary interventions for financial gain that could have negative medical outcomes in this healthy woman.

Identifying the source of her anxiety as social pressure will likely help this patient to deal with it. Providing examples of couples who took longer to get pregnant, and did so without intervention may be reassuring. Building trust, providing support and indicating understanding of her dilemma would probably be the best safeguard against her doctor shopping.

Case study III: Abuse toward the wife

Layla comes in with several broken bones. Upon interview, she reports that her husband is possessed by an angry spirit, and she has gone to religious healers to have him cured.

Analysis

Layla is being physically abused by her husband. Psychosocial issues may or may not be addressed through the extended family. This should be handled sensitively, as many people do not want to talk about these types of issues with "strangers". While many people believe that marrying within the family will protect the wife, this is not always the case. In some cases, the extended family can help effectively in dealing with this type of violence. In other cases where violence has become routine in the family, the family will not be helpful. Also, Layla's case may only be the "tip of the iceberg". Many women who are physically or emotionally abused are reluctant to disclose this fact, and come to the health center with numerous vague complaints that are not amenable to diagnosis or treatment. A great deal of morbidity in the primary care setting worldwide is due to hidden emotional or social factors. Some clinics in various countries employ special staff dedicated to recognizing domestic abuse and to helping women.

Case study IV: Young daughter with depression

Maryam, aged 16, comes to the clinic with her mother, because she has experienced severe weight loss and lack of appetite. Her mother insists on staying with Maryam, so the doctor cannot interview Maryam alone. Her mother appears very upset when the doctor asks questions related to psychological issues.

Analysis

Family versus individual

Maryam sees herself as part of her family, not as an individual person. Her mother feels that she is supporting her daughter by staying with her all the time, and is anxious about the idea of leaving Maryam alone, especially with a male doctor. She cannot imagine that there is anything that Maryam would want to say privately to a "stranger" (the doctor). There are times when family support is very helpful, and other times when it can be a burden. The doctor should not assume that either is the case but remain alert to the patient's concerns.

The social stigma against mental illness

Maryam and her mother are worried about what people will say if they find out that Maryam's weight loss is due to a psychiatric condition. What if this damages Maryam's prospects in her community?

There is a lot of social stigma against psychiatric illness. The family should understand that everyone is vulnerable to psychiatric illness, and that depression is very common and is curable with counseling and perhaps medication. Like other physical diseases, it can be treated without permanently affecting the person's identity. The family can be informed about what to expect and what they can do to support their daughter. They should not assume that it is due to a "lack of faith" or that there is something or someone specific who is to blame. For example, the mother should not think that she is a bad parent because her daughter has depression. They can be educated that spiritual and religious counsel can be sought in addition to medical treatment.

Case study V: Woman seeking contraception

A woman comes to the clinic wanting contraception, but her husband is against it.

Analysis

The practitioner should attempt to understand what exactly the husband is objecting to, and why the woman wants the contraception. They may be able to settle their issues with a counselor or family member. It may be that the woman is exhausted from her current work and care of her children and does not receive enough support in the family. It may be that the husband is concerned about side-effects of the contraceptive. The husband may be under social pressure from his family to produce more children. Studies from Egypt have demonstrated that involving husbands during antenatal visits can be effective in improving contraceptive uptake rates in the postpartum period.[4] It may be helpful to inform the husband of the benefits of pregnancy spacing on the children's health.

Case study VI: Telling bad news

Amir is 26 years old and has been diagnosed with leukemia. He has a poor prognosis. His parents do not want the doctor to tell him his diagnosis.

Analysis

In many European countries and in the United States, the primary emphasis in clinical practice is on the patient's individualism or "autonomy". However, people in many cultures and communities prefer a more family-centered approach to decision-making. The patient and family's preferences in this case should be seen in the context of how they lived in the past. An individual who consulted closely with family about other important life decisions – such as the choice of a mate, a career, and the names of his children – would likely prefer to trust in his family to share or take on the burden of making critical decisions during times of crisis.

Families often do not want the patient to know a poor prognosis. This partially reflects beliefs about the power of hope, and the negative consequences on the individual of losing hope. The family feels that the patient may be better able to recover if he believes he can. This may also represent a symbolic "lightening the load" on the patient by insisting that the family take on the burden of knowledge of the poor prognosis. Frequently in clinical practice, the patient, especially if he or she is well educated, has at least some knowledge of the prognosis but often conceals this from the family. Perhaps this "mutual protection" pattern echoes familiar socially encouraged models of self-sacrifice for other family members. Through knowledge of the family, and careful history-taking, both patient and family needs can frequently be accommodated in the clinical setting. However, much more research needs to be carried out on this topic in the Arab world.

As demonstrated in the above case scenarios, there are many aspects of medical practice that need further study from a cultural perspective. Exploring medical topics from a cultural perspective may illustrate how a different approach or model may be required for optimal understanding of these issues in different cultures.

The meaning of illness

Medical anthropologists have focused on the various meanings of "illness", "health" and what counts as "normal" in different societies. For example, the medical diagnosis of infertility impacts women in Arab societies differently than it does women in Euro-American societies. Whereas in American society, many couples may choose to be childless, in Arab society one can usually assume that a childless couple suffers from infertility. The social and cultural impact of infertility on women is particularly acute, such that childless women are viewed, and often consider themselves, as "incomplete". This is an example of the ways in which a single condition – infertility – may be experienced differently in different social and cultural environments, and the ways in which different social environments differentially define what it is to be "normal".

Studies in the United States have explored the cultural contexts of different populations, and have contributed to the provision of improved healthcare by uncovering cultural obstacles to treatment. In one example from the 1960s, medical anthropologists studied neonatal intensive care units in the United States and assessed that the isolation of premature babies from their mothers for extended periods of time (for fear of the premature infants becoming "infected" outside the sterile environment of their ward) led to depression in mothers and failure to thrive in infants. In many cases, the new mothers abandoned the infants from whom they were separated. Following the results of this study, protocols for neonatal care were modified to encourage interaction between mother and infant. The physicians found that, contrary to the assumption that the infants would become infected outside the sterile environment, they were actually more likely to thrive with increased maternal contact.

In this example, orthodox medical thinking fostered a cultural value in which "sterility" was more important than "mother–infant interaction". This assumption prevented the best possible care for these infants. It is important to study exactly how different cultural norms are established in the medical profession and how these norms are received and interpreted by different patient groups. For example, by using American and European medical texts and other resources, medical professionals in the Arab world benefit by being able to access a large quantity of diverse, up-to-date and high-quality medical information. Yet a disadvantage is that much of this literature is based on populations living in vastly different social, economic and cultural situations. This may encourage some healthcare providers to unconsciously internalize assumptions, practices and expectations toward health and appropriate management of certain medical problems that may not be warranted, given their own settings. This phenomenon is not limited to healthcare professionals. Patients and others are often influenced by the media or other sources to believe that certain Western practices, treatments or lifestyles are "better" or "more advanced" regardless of whether they are or not.

Genetic counseling

When medical interventions developed in one region are introduced into another, successful application of these practices often depends on certain resources and conditions being present in the recipient community. These include material resources but ìn may in addition involve social attitudes, habits and worldviews.

For example, in the United States and Europe, genetic counseling is available to many groups and individuals who are at risk for genetic diseases. Individuals who may be carrying genes for certain diseases are tested, as are their spouses. If testing reveals a significant risk of transmission of disease to a child that might be conceived by the couple, they are counseled and allowed to make their own decision as to whether or not to proceed with having children. Medical, ethical and practical guidelines for genetic counseling and management have been developed in Western countries and have been shown to reduce the burden of genetic disease in populations affected by high rates of genetic illnesses. Attempts to apply these practices in Arab countries, however, have met with mixed results. This may be due to very different perceptions, priorities and traditions among families and communities in the Arab world.[5,6] Whereas genetic counseling as conventionally practiced has been designed in a culture where decisions such as marriage and fertility are often narrowly based on individual priorities, in many Arab communities, matters of marriage and procreation tend to involve the family and community. This is illustrated by a report of a genetic counseling intervention in a Bedouin family from the Negev desert. Studies identified some family members as carriers of a hereditary metabolic disease. After family members received counseling, many of the men broke tradition and married outside the family. The unmarried women of the family were stigmatized in the community and subsequently married as second or third wives to other close family members. In addition to the social problems this caused, the genetic burden of illness in the family was unchanged.[7] Other studies have suggested that individuals and families might respond to genetic counseling programs in unexpected ways, such as those attempting to use the information to gain advantage in marriage negotiations.[8] This highlights the importance of carefully studying traditional and societal values, and designing modifications to ensure that interventions are congruent with community practices and expectations. This is another illustration of the fact that communities are rarely entirely passive in their acceptance of new medical interventions.

The end of life

By focusing on social and cultural factors in medical practice, we may find that certain practices that are taken to be medical or scientific "facts" in one area are not accepted as such universally. For example, recent work has provided a detailed analysis of why clinical death, or brain death, has been accepted as medical "fact" in North America for the past two decades but was rejected in Japan. While both Japan and North America have highly sophisticated medical technology, different social experiences of death led to different medical practices surrounding what is clearly not purely a medical question. Death is both a biological and social process, and yet modern institutions mark it as a particular concrete event. North American medical practitioners were able to assume control over re-defining "death" so that it changed from the old definition (namely as the end of cardio-pulmonary function) to a new one (the end of cortical function). However, in Japan, families and medical practitioners did not accept the cessation of brain function as the end of life as long as patients' cardiopulmonary status was preserved. This study demonstrated that a particular technology (such as the concept of brain death) is not always readily transportable from one context to another.[9]

Bioethics

Another area in medicine that may deserve scrutiny is the field of bioethics. Bioethics often presents itself as a universal discipline, despite the fact that it is dominated by the tenets and assumptions of Western philosophical, "rationalistic" thought and regional historical events.[10] Within the purview of bioethics are topics such as patient confidentiality, truth, informed consent in medical treatment and experimentation, definitions of personhood, withholding or withdrawing life-sustaining treatments, and the ownership and transplantation of body parts and genetic materials.[11] Many scholars have questioned bioethicists' tendencies to define such concepts as "beneficence" or "harm" across the globe without adequately taking into consideration cultural or historic differences.

Besides the problem of ethnocentricity, the bioethics concept of "society" may require scrutiny. For example, it was assumed in the United States that the introduction of technologies for prenatal diagnostic testing would reduce the burden of genetic disease. The assumption was that if pregnant women tested positively for carrying a fetus with a genetic disease, such as Down syndrome, these woman would elect to end the pregnancy. However, women did not always make this choice and indeed came to very different decisions about their test results. The ways in which women defined a "healthy" pregnancy varied, depending either on social factors such as their socioeconomic status, ethnicity, religious background or family relations or on their past experiences with physical or mental disabilities.[12]

This study, which highlighted a plurality of perspectives, refuted the standard bioethical concept of "society" as if it were a homogenous, discrete unit. Although many genetic counselors assumed that a woman would undergo abortion when informed of a fetal abnormality, they found that this was not always the case. This demonstrates that different people have different opinions about what counts as "worthy life".

Organ transplantation

Another study explored bioethical issues surrounding organ transplantation in a Muslim society in Egypt.[13] This study suggested that even within the same cultural, religious and socioeconomic group, there can be vastly differing opinions about a particular medical practice.

Unlike the situation outlined above, in which individuals in the United States had no single, agreed set of ethical guidelines to follow, the members of a Muslim society are in general agreement about a set of ethical guidelines to follow – namely the Islamic primary texts; the Holy Qur'an and the Sunna. However, as we know, agreement on a single source of ethical authority does not mean that all Muslims will behave in exactly the same way when faced with a life-or-death situation. Some issues are clearer than others. For example, there is no controversy about the ethics of active euthanasia, or what is referred to as "mercy killing". From an Islamic viewpoint, it is simply forbidden for a physician to actively end a patient's life in order to end his suffering, regardless of the wishes of the patient. Here the Qur'anic injunctions against suicide and murder clearly override the bioethical value of patient autonomy. This is different from the patient's wish to withdraw from or end treatment, which is considered permissible by many scholars.

In the case of organ transplants, in-depth interviews were conducted with physicians, patients and their families to try to understand why many renal failure patients refused to consider kidney transplant as an option for them, despite their physician's encouragement to do so. Several patients explained their reluctance in religious terms, saying that God is the sole Healer, and that the whole body and its parts belong to God alone, and it is not the human's right to interfere with them. This argument was advanced by many patients despite *fatawa* from Sheikh al Azhar and other Islamic scholars permitting organ transplant under conditions of necessity; benefit to the recipient, lack of harm to the donor, and the absence of any commercial transaction.

The patients in this study felt that dialysis was a very difficult process but one that they could endure. Many spoke of their constant vulnerability to infection during dialysis sessions. They also had their own explanation of the etiology of their disease. Although the cause of their kidney failure was recorded by their physicians as "unknown" or "idiopathic", many patients insisted that the cause of their kidney failure was environmental. For example, they cited such factors as contamination of the water, pesticides in vegetables, hormone injections in chickens, chemical fertilizers and other types of "unnatural" pollutants.

These Muslim patients, when asked why they did not consider organ transplants, replied that it was because they believed it was "*haram*", despite the fact that their Muslim physicians did not hold this same view. Through questioning and spending time with these patients, one can understand the social-cultural background informing the different viewpoints of patients and physicians. Both patients and physicians agreed that Islam was the sole source of ethical guidance in these decisions. Furthermore, patients and the physicians also agreed on the basic Islamic principles: that God is the sole Healer (*al-Shafi*), that all sickness and all cure comes from God alone, that no patient should be submitted to harm, and that treatment should be sought in case of sickness. If all agreed with these tenets, then why did they have different decisions regarding organ transplants?

Understanding the social circumstances and cognitive processes of both patients and physicians reveals the answer to this question. Patients who were reluctant to consider organ transplant feared harming their spouses or siblings by "taking" a kidney from them. One patient, a young man in his late twenties, refused many times his wife's offer to donate her kidney to him. He said: "It is bad enough that one of us is sick, why should I make her sick with me?" This patient, like many others, believed that the environment in which he lived made him vulnerable to sickness and ultimately led to his kidney failure. He believed that if he were to cause his wife to live in this same environment with only one kidney, then he would be increasing her chances of being sick also. Additionally, this patient, like many others, feared that his wife might not withstand the stress of an operation. His previous experiences with the medical profession (in which he had been misdiagnosed several times before the realization that he needed dialysis) led him to mistrust doctors, fear hospitals and avoid the risk of submitting his wife to the same health issues from which he himself suffered. Furthermore, he would constantly say that he was grateful to God for his dialysis treatment. As long as he was able to withstand the dialysis sessions, he did not see the need of putting his family at risk, harming his wife and submitting himself to an operation of which the result, as he pointed out, was not "guaranteed". "God is the sole Guarantor" he would repeatedly say.

This case example helps explain why this particular Muslim patient refused to consider organ transplant. The medical staff attending to him assumed that the reason for his refusal was simply the high financial cost of the operation or perhaps the patient's ignorance and his misguided belief that the operation was *haram*. Yet anthropological methodology, which aims to understand the social circumstances which help to form the patient's decisions, suggests that this patient was not, in fact, ignorant. He used sound Islamic ethical reasoning to support his decision – indeed the same reasoning that the physicians used to support the use of organ transplant. The points in which they differ do not turn on Islamic principles but rather on their different interpretations of the nature of the organ transplant itself. The physicians believe that the operation will not harm the donor, while the patient believes that it will. The physicians believe that the operation will be to the benefit of the patient, while the patient is not assured that this is the case. The physicians believe that the organ transplant is a necessity and that dialysis is not the best option for this young patient, while the patient himself feels that as long as he is doing well on dialysis, there is no necessity for a transplant. Finally, the physicians believe that the patient's kidney failure is specific to that particular patient, while the patient believes that there is a high risk of the environment causing kidney failure, to which his wife will be doubly exposed if she were to donate her kidney to him. This case suggests the importance of understanding patients' social circumstances and beliefs about the etiology of their disease, the nature of the medical intervention, and their previous experiences with the medical profession. Medical practitioners should be certain that the patient understands risks and benefits of procedures from the medical perspective, but should respect the patient's own consideration of these risks in terms of other factors as well. Such factors might include their family's economic resources and their own personal beliefs and experiential knowledge.

In conclusion, the study of culture has many applications to the practice of medicine in the Arab world. First, we can identify particular historical or social factors that have helped to shape medical practice. Also important is the identification of social factors contributing to patients' and physicians' ethical decision-making. If we agree on the bioethical principle of self-determination or autonomy, yet at the same time wish to offer the patient the best choices for his or her well-being and treatment, then we must be able to understand the patient's social contexts which are contingent on these principles. Finally, the study of culture can provide analyses of how the same medical practice or technology can be received differently in different places or by different people. A specific medical practice or technology that is invented and designed for a particular context will not necessarily have the same effects in different contexts. Historically, models of health, illness and therapy in the Arab world have been dominated by Western constructs. This is not surprising, given the disparity in resources and research between the two geographic regions. Healthcare professionals and scientists in the Arab world should begin to explore, develop and integrate local models of health and disease into education and practice while remaining aware of the dynamism and diversity of human culture.

References

1 Al-Qutob R, Mawajdeh S, Allosh R *et al.* The effect of prenatal knowledge of fetal sex on birth weight: a study from Jordan. *Health Care Women Int* 2004; **25 (3):** 281–91.

2 El-Mehairy T. *Medical Doctors: a study of role concept and job satisfaction: the Egyptian case.* Leiden: EJ Brill; 1984.

3 Al-Mutlak H, Chaleby K. Group psychotherapy with Arab patients. *Arab Journal of Psychiatry* 1995; **6 (2):** 125–36.

4 Soliman MH. Impact of antenatal counselling on couples' knowledge and practice of contraception in Mansoura, Egypt. *East Mediterr Health J* 1999; **5 (5):** 1002–13.

5 Bayoumi RA, Yardumian A. Genetic disease in the Arab world. *BMJ* 2006; **333 (7573):** 819.

6 Al-Gazali LI. Attitudes toward genetic counseling in the United Arab Emirates. *Community Genet* 2005; **8 (1):** 48–51.

7 Carmi R, Elbedour K, Wietzman D *et al.* Lowering the burden of hereditary diseases in a traditional, inbred community: ethical aspects of genetic research and its application. *Sci Context* 1998; **11 (3–4):** 391–5.

8 Raz A, Atar M. Upright generations of the future: tradition and medicalization in community genetics. *Journal of Contemporary Ethnography* 2004; **33 (3):** 296–322.

9 Lock MM. *Twice Dead: organ transplants and the reinvention of death.* Berkeley: University of California Press; 2002.

10 Borry P, Schotsmans P, Dierickx K. How international is bioethics? A quantitative retrospective study. *BMC Med Ethics* 2006; **7 (1):** E1.

11 Marshall PA. Anthropology and bioethics. *Med Anthropol Q* 1992; **6 (1):** 49–73.

12 Rapp R. *Testing Women, Testing the Fetus: the social impact of amniocentesis in America.* New York: Routledge; 1999.

13 Hamdy S. *Our Bodies Belong to God: Islam, medical science, and ethical reasoning in Egyptian life.* New York: New York University; 2006.

CHAPTER 2

Globalization, health and culture

(★ *Laeth S Nasir*

Introduction

Globalization has been defined as economic processes that are characterized by increasing international integration of markets for goods, services and capital.[1] Alternatively, it has been described as a process in which the traditional boundaries that have separated societies and communities recede.[2] With the growing prevalence and reach of these processes, complex changes are occurring worldwide, both in national economies and, to an increasing degree, in culture, politics, and ultimately health and health behavior. A great deal of debate has been stirred by this issue; both from those who feel that the international economic and cultural order is threatened by globalization, and from those who argue that economic and technological integration are key to solving the problems of the world's poor.[1] Regardless of the outcome of this argument, it is clear that the ongoing changes that are taking place are having profound impacts on families and communities throughout the world. Because of this, understanding the connection between these changes and their potential effects on the health of populations and individuals is critical for healthcare providers and planners.

This chapter will briefly review some of the changes that these processes may have on the health of populations and individuals in Arab countries.

Broad determinants of health

Many of the changes initiated by globalization are not introduced into cultural and historical voids; rather, they take place in regions that have their own local history, dynamics, customs and traditions. Therefore, rather than being purely "Westernizing" or "homogenizing" they tend to have complex effects on societies whose ultimate outcomes are often difficult to predict.

The complexity of the relationships between globalization, social and mental well-being and overall health are only recently beginning to be understood.[2] Many of these links are mediated through what have been termed the "broad determinants of health" by some authors.[3] These determinants include social, environmental and biological factors that have been found to correlate with health status.

Primarily social factors

- *income and social status:* these include economic resources and the position within a society that an individual holds. In general, the poor are less healthy than the rich, due to factors such as nutrition and access to healthcare.
- *education:* high educational attainment is related to better employment prospects, more secure employment, and better access to healthcare.
- *social support networks:* access to strong social support from community, friends and family is associated with improved health, particularly mental health.
- *employment:* employed individuals are generally healthier than the unemployed. Secure employment and good working conditions are important determinants of health status.
- *personal health practices and coping skills:* these include hygiene, diet, activity, smoking and other substance use, as well as sexual behaviors.
- *culture:* health beliefs, dietary and other customs, traditions, value systems and moral codes of societies have important effects on the patterns and types of illnesses seen in a given culture or region.

Primarily environmental factors

- *the physical environment:* safe working conditions, clean water and a safe food supply are important contributors to health at both the individual and population levels.
- *health services:* the availability of accessible, good quality healthcare is important in the prevention and treatment of disease, at both individual and community levels.

Primarily biological factors

- *gender:* patterns of diseases differ between genders. This is due to biological factors as well as cultural expectations, roles and pressures that are experienced differentially according to gender.
- *genetics:* an individual's genetic endowment is an important determinant of health status and health outcomes.

Effects of globalization on economies

Both promoters and detractors of the processes of globalization agree that globalization impacts many factors that influence the broad determinants of health. The primary disagreement is whether or not the changes deliver a net health benefit to people in different parts of the world.

Work

The processes of globalization have had important effects on the types of work available and the availability of jobs in many regions. Some areas have experienced increased worker incomes. These changes may improve health by translating into better household nutrition, sanitation and education. In response, there has been growing migration from rural to urban areas. This may result in changes in population make-up of some areas. For example, one study of Bedouin populations in the Bekaa Valley in Lebanon reported significant changes in women's occupations and responsibilities to fill the void left by the outmigration of young men from their communities to the cities.[4]

Increasingly, work is being "informalized" and "delocalized" through the creation of jobs that are temporary. The rewards of higher household incomes that may lead to improvements in health due to better healthcare, nutrition and living conditions might be tempered over the long term by increased stress due to the family and community disruption that results from increased mobility.

Women's workforce participation

Although women's rates of participation in the labor force are lower in Arab countries than most other areas of the world, these rates are growing rapidly as a result of globalizing forces.[5] Changes in gender make-up of the workforce may have many interconnected effects. The conventional notion is that increased formal workforce participation translates into increased income for women; and that this improves women's social status. It is likely, however, that the dynamics of this process are more complex than this simple formula would suggest. For example, working women may have to delay childbearing or limit their fertility due to increased work responsibilities, and some jobs may represent a hazard to their childbearing function.[6] Among some groups, a large number of children may be a woman's only acceptable option for social status and long-term security.[7] Domestic responsibilities, which have traditionally been assigned to women, including childcare and care of the elderly or disabled, may be proportionately neglected, leading to feelings of guilt and social conflict. In addition, the cost of obtaining child or elder care may reduce the financial gain expected through employment. Often, women are expected to continue much of the traditionally mandated household and childcare duties in addition to their employment. This may create a double burden for them and subsequently increase mental health problems and stress-related illness, as two studies from Egypt suggest.[8,9]

One study from Jordan explored the intensity of perceived stress, and physical symptoms reported by women who worked for a wage and those who did not. The study found that working women tended to report less perceived stress than those who did not work, but the statistical power of this study was not robust. It was also noted that the research instrument may not have accurately reflected the nature of stressors experienced in Arab culture.[10] Another study in Jordan found that work stress was a small but significant contributing factor to depressive symptoms among women in a primary care setting.[11]

Education

The characteristics of the globalized economy are also resulting in changes in the nature of work. Academic institutions face challenges in modifying their curricula, as the skills and educational quality of graduates may not match the needs of the rapidly changing work environment. This may result in increased unemployment and unmet expectations among youth.

Healthcare

Tasks such as healthcare and provision of utilities that traditionally have been the responsibility of governments may be increasingly shifted to the private sector. This often results in increases in efficiency and cost savings, but may also shift excessive cost burdens to families and individuals, thereby reducing access to healthcare or essential utilities.[12] Prices and availability of pharmaceuticals may also be affected by international agreements and market forces as cost controls are lifted.[13]

Challenges to governments include ensuring that the economic benefits of globalization translate into overall health benefits to the population. This requires management and oversight to ensure that any economic growth is sustainable, and that the long-term social, economic and environmental effects of new policies on local culture are understood before these changes are put into place.

Environmental issues

The connections between globalization and environmental change are poorly studied, as in the case of the spread of communicable disease. At the simplest level, the extraordinary mobility of populations and goods may lead to outbreaks of communicable diseases in distant corners the world.[14] One example of this was the unprecedented speed with which the spread of severe acute respiratory syndrome (SARS) occurred internationally. Unfamiliar illnesses may be spread to new areas that are poorly prepared to deal with them.[15] These have included diseases such as human immuno-deficiency virus (HIV) or tuberculosis but may also include agricultural or other pests that might threaten a country's agricultural infrastructure or wildlife.

Among other important health threats are the often unplanned urbanization in areas experiencing rapid population increases. This growth can place severe strains on government health, social and educational budgets and services, and may result in problems with crowding and sanitation.

Modernization of urban areas may take place in ways that result in unhealthy outcomes. For example, in many areas, urban growth may proceed with little regard for the social, physical or mental health of residents.[16,17] The absence of pedestrian facilities often results in an excessive dependence on cars or other transport, leading to air pollution, sedentary lifestyles and obesity.[18] Features such as widely dispersed housing, or apartment blocks, and poorly planned neighborhoods, often lead to artificial separation of families and communities, an absence of areas for recreation, less socialization and support, and consequently an increase in social and psychological problems.[19]

Cultural issues

Cultural change may result in individual and community level changes in health behavior. This may lead to new patterns of health risk developing in the region. For example, mass education and international education may give rise to expectations among youth, particularly among women, that diverge from traditional roles.[20,21] Media such as film and satellite television are already resulting in much cultural change, particularly among youth who, as a result of having more exposure to these media, are developing different expectations than their parents' generation. These differences in attitudes have been shown to cause an increase in psychiatric symptoms in families[22] and are often expressed through increased consumerism, material expectations and changes in ethnic identity. Community reaction to this phenomenon may include the rising popularity of organized religion and increased emphasis on traditional marriage patterns.

Marketing of Western-style foods may also result in dietary change, leading to increased intakes of calorie-dense food, reductions in vegetable and fruit consumption and subsequent increases in obesity related morbidity.[23,24] Tobacco is an important cause of illness and death among adults in Arab countries. In addition, globalization has increased illicit cross-border flows of populations, drugs and people.

Populations displaced because of violence and political instability also suffer from increased social and mental health problems, due to the loss of traditional community support systems as well as to crowding and competition for housing, jobs and food.[25] Refugee populations tend to have very high rates of mental health problems, including depression, anxiety and post-traumatic stress disorder.[26,27]

Solutions to many of the problems brought about by these complex issues will depend on the development of creative research agendas and policies that will anticipate and respond to these challenges by leveraging the strengths inherent in Arab culture. Successfully meeting these changes with integrity and innovation will be critical in determining the future of our children and societies.

References

1 Dollar D. Is globalization good for your health? *Bull World Health Organ* 2001; **79 (9):** 827–32.

2 Bhugra D, Mastrogianni A. Globalisation and mental disorders: overview with relation to depression. *Br J Psychiatry* 2004; **184:** 10–20.

3 Yach D. "Health-for-all" in the twenty-first century: a global perspective. *Natl Med J India* 1997; **10 (2):** 82–9.

4 Guest G. *Globalization, Health, and the Environment: an integrated perspective.* Lanham, MD: AltaMira Press; 2005.

5 Sidani Y. Women, work, and Islam in Arab societies. *Women in Management Review* 2005; **20 (7):** 498–512.

6 Taha TE, Gray RH. Agricultural pesticide exposure and perinatal mortality in central Sudan. *Bull World Health Organ* 1993; **71 (3–4):** 317–21.

7 Fahim HI, Faris R. Child abuse as an inhibiting factor for family planning. *J Egypt Public Health Assoc* 1992; **67 (1–2):** 1–11.

8 Hattar-Pollara M, Meleis AI, Nagib H. A study of the spousal role of Egyptian women in clerical jobs. *Health Care Women Int* 2000; **21 (4):** 305–17.

9 Hattar-Pollara M, Meleis AI, Nagib H. Multiple role stress and patterns of coping of Egyptian women in clerical jobs. *J Transcult Nurs* 2003; **14 (2):** 125–33.

10 Hattar-Pollara M, Dawani H. Cognitive appraisal of stress and health status of wage working and non-wage working women in Jordan. *J Transcult Nurs* 2006; **17 (4):** 349–56.

11 Hamid H, Abu-Hijleh NS, Sharif SL *et al.* A primary care study of the correlates of depressive symptoms among Jordanian women. *Transcult Psychiatry* 2004; **41 (4):** 487–96.

12 Woodward D, Drager N, Beaglehole R *et al.* Globalization and health: a framework for analysis and action. *Bull World Health Organ* 2001; **79 (9):** 875–81.

13 Khoja TA, Bawazir SA. Group purchasing of pharmaceuticals and medical supplies by the Gulf Cooperation Council states. *East Mediterr Health J* 2005; **11 (1–2):** 217–25.

14 Bygbjerg IC, Krasnik A. The global fight against diseases – a race against time. *Dan Med Bull* 2007; **54 (1):** 31.

15 Smith R, Woodward D, Acharya A *et al.* Communicable disease control: a "Global Public Good" perspective. *Health Policy Plan* 2004; **19 (5):** 271–8.

16 Chaix B, Rosvall M, Merlo J. Assessment of the magnitude of geographical variations and socioeconomic contextual effects on ischaemic heart disease mortality: a multilevel survival analysis of a large Swedish cohort. *J Epidemiol Community Health* 2007; **61 (4):** 349–55.

17 Semenza JC, March TL, Bontempo BD. Community-initiated urban development: an ecological intervention. *J Urban Health* 2007; **84 (1):** 8–20.

18 Kochtitzky CS, Frumkin H, Rodriguez R *et al.* Urban planning and public health at CDC. *MMWR Morb Mortal Wkly Rep* 2006; **55 Suppl 2:** 34–8.

19 Guite HF, Clark C, Ackrill G. The impact of the physical and urban environment on mental well-being. *Public Health* 2006; **120 (12):** 1117–26.

20 Schvaneveldt P, Kerpelman J, Schvaneveldt J. Generational and cultural changes in family life in the United Arab Emirates: a comparison of mothers and daughters. *Journal of Comparative Family Studies* 2005; **36 (1):** 77–91.

21 Almutawa M. Values change and its effects on women status in the UAE society: comparative field study on a sample of educated working and non-working women. *Journal of the Social Sciences* 2002; **30 (2):** 347–79.

22 El-Islam MF. Interparental differences in attitudes to cultural changes in Kuwait. *Soc Psychiatry Psychiatr Epidemiol* 1988; **23:** 109–13.

23 Bashour HN. Survey of dietary habits of in-school adolescents in Damascus, Syrian Arab Republic. *East Mediterr Health J* 2004; **10 (6):** 853–62.

24 Malik M, Bakir A. Prevalence of overweight and obesity among children in the United Arab Emirates. *Obes Rev* 2007; **8 (1):** 15–20.

25 Burnett A. Globalization, migration and health. *Med Confl Surviv* 2002; **18 (1):** 34–43.

26 Jamil H, Hakim-Larson J, Farrag M *et al.* A retrospective study of Arab American mental health clients: trauma and the Iraqi refugees. *Am J Orthopsychiatry* 2002; **72 (3):** 355–61.

27 Momartin S, Steel Z, Coello M *et al.* A comparison of the mental health of refugees with temporary versus permanent protection visas. *Med J Aust* 2006; **185 (7):** 357–61.

CHAPTER 3

Gender and health

(★ *Laeth S Nasir and Raeda Al-Qutob*

Introduction

Women's health has been understudied historically. Only recently has the medical field begun to examine many of the more subtle differences in healthcare needs between men and women, and considered many of the biological, social and cultural factors that affect the sexes differentially.

When examining disparities between the sexes, it is important to understand the social dynamics that affect gender and health in a contextual fashion. Researchers and practitioners should appreciate the reciprocal roles that men and women play in society, and how these roles impact the health of both sexes. In the Arab world, women's roles are rapidly changing in many areas. This creates both opportunities to improve health, as well as dangers of exposure to new health hazards.

Addressing women's health issues is important in the public health setting because of the disproportionate impact that they have on the health of the larger community. Women not only comprise 50% of the population, but they also bear a disproportionate share of health problems, primarily as a result of their childbearing role. In addition, women are primarily responsible for the health and well-being of their children. Women further provide most of the care for the old and the disabled in a population. Therefore, strategies that optimize the health of women and girls, particularly those emphasizing education, have been shown to dramatically improve the health of populations in other parts of the world.[1] Although there are few studies that explore these effects in the Arab world, studies do exist that demonstrate that the incidence of developmental delay is much lower among the offspring of educated women compared to those having less education.[2,3]

This chapter will focus on a range of issues that affect the health of women in the Arab world. It should be kept in mind that literature reviews, studies and other scientific works that explore many of these issues in Arab countries are relatively scarce; therefore, much remains to be done in terms of performing studies and developing theoretical constructs to capture the complete picture.

Sociocultural determinants of health

It has long been known that gender is one of the major determinants of health conditions that will be experienced by individuals and populations (*see also* Chapter 2, Globalization, health and culture). The reasons for this are not just biological but also involve sociocultural, religious, political and economic factors. Sociocultural factors include value judgments made by families and societies regarding the relative worth and position of individuals, depending on their gender. These forces may result in the differential distribution of material and emotional resources based on gender. The disparity in literacy rates between men and women in Arab countries is only one of the most visible manifestations of this inequity.[4]

Political factors can also have significant impacts on health. Policies and programs often affect men and women differently. In many Arab countries, the low numbers of decision-makers in health systems who are women may contribute to a lack of policies and programs that are uniformly suited to the needs of both genders.

Whether arising primarily from society, culture or government, these factors impact health at many levels. These include whether an individual decides to seek healthcare for themselves or a member of their family, the barriers that they may encounter in seeking care, and the appropriateness, quality and outcome of care that is obtained.

Gender, gender preference and health

Prevailing social attitudes regarding gender have been reported to occur as early as the antenatal period. One study from Jordan reported that pregnant women who had prenatal knowledge of their baby's sex through ultrasound delivered significantly heavier males than those who were not informed of the baby's sex. Presumably, this difference was due to conscious or unconscious efforts on the part of the mother and/or her family to optimize maternal nutrition and prenatal care.[5] In Egypt, women married to illiterate husbands were ten times more likely to express desire for a son than those married to more educated men.[6] Negative maternal emotional states and obstetric difficulties were reported among Egyptian women pregnant with a child antenatally identified as being of the undesired sex.[7] A baby's female sex was an independent risk factor for low birth weight in a study from Saudi Arabia.[8] One study from Syria showed that male children were significantly more likely to be taken to medical visits than females.[9] Also in Egypt, gender differences in child mortality were reported to diminish with increasing maternal educational level.[10]

Data on the extent of sex preference in the medical literature are mixed, however. One study examining healthcare behavior in Tunisia and Morocco found smaller than expected gender differences in several measures of healthcare.[11] Some authors report that the extent of gender preference varies from region to region, being greatest in the Levant and Gulf regions, and less marked in North Africa.[12]

Marriage and health

Marriage is a major social institution forming the family in Arab society.

Communal and family interests have traditionally played a major role in marriage in Arab culture. Practices such as arranged marriage and consanguineous unions have reflected the close involvement of family and community in every aspect of the life of the individual. This shared commitment provides critical ongoing social, economic and moral support to the new family, and propagates family interdependency and cohesion.

Traditionally, courtship and marriage behaviors among all faith traditions in the region were subject to rigid cultural norms. In the past, arranged marriages were the rule. Parents or other interested relatives would act as agents to represent the interests of both individuals involved as well as the families concerned.

More recently, the norm for marriage has been shifting to a more individualistic pattern, and a less prominent family role, particularly in the middle and upper classes. However, in general, the final selection of a mate is still made in close consultation with family members. This is illustrated by continued strong religious and group endogamy in marriage patterns.[13] The degree of independence of mate selection among women seems to be strengthened by increased education[14] and generational change.[15,16] One study reported that the degree of autonomy in selection of a mate was positively correlated with self-perceived marital quality, although the methodology used was questionable.[17]

Marriage

Marriage in all cultures is considered a joyful transition. However, the process of forming a new family unit, with its changing alliances, living conditions and, frequently, its new geographical location, is often very stressful – particularly if the individuals involved are young, and have little experience of life outside their own families. It is at this point that many practitioners may see conditions due to anxiety or lack of preparation of one partner or both of the married couple. One author describes a subset of young women who anticipate or experience failure to cope with early married life, and who develop emotionally generated somatic symptoms that result in their inability to marry or fulfil their marital role.[18] Another describes "nuptial psychosis" – a stress-induced dissociative or psychotic state occurring in young brides who are poorly prepared for marriage.[19] One report from Jordan explored the experiences of 116 couples referred for psychiatric care with a complaint of unconsummated marriage and in whom an organic cause had been excluded. The majority of subjects were reported to be between the ages of 20 and 29. Risk factors for inability to consummate the marriage were reported to include poor education, an arranged marriage, the bride having to move away from her family, and pressure from the family for proof of consummation.[20] A study from Saudi Arabia that compared 39 couples referred for unconsummated marriage with 37 controls found no significant differences between couples regarding the acquisition of sexual information, education or avocation. However, wives in the affected group were more likely to be young and display high sexual anxiety. Vaginismus and erectile dysfunction were common. It was reported that 87% of the couples believed that supernatural influences were to blame.[21] Awareness by the physician of the upcoming marital transition, monitoring anxiety, and counseling the young couple and family, may be important interventions to reduce the degree of stress experienced by all involved parties.

Sexuality

Attitudes toward sexuality and reproduction are formed in childhood, and transmitted across generations.[22] Traditional attitudes toward sexuality are strongly protective against such reproductive health risks as sexually transmitted diseases (STDs), and out-of-wedlock births. On the other hand, taboos around these subjects tend to inhibit access to information about sexual and reproductive health. Although some data suggest that, particularly for young girls, parents are the preferred source of information on sex and sexuality,[23] it has been noted that parents are often poorly prepared to advise their children on sexual matters.[24] This observation is supported by studies from several countries reporting widespread ignorance among adolescents regarding normal pubertal development.[23-5] Some authorities report that the anxiety engendered by some parents' and families' efforts to educate their children, particularly females, about sexual matters may result in excessive anxiety with sexual contact or low sexual desire, with negative consequences after marriage.[26,27]

Because of the taboo on discussions of sexuality, complaints regarding sexual problems in married couples often present to the physician as marital conflict. Later, it may be discovered that the actual difficulty is sexual in nature. Published reports of sexual dysfunction from the Arab world focus primarily on male sexual dysfunction. Authorities state that it is very rare for women to present with problems related to sexual health, such as low desire or orgasmic dysfunction. When female dysfunction does come to medical attention, it is usually in the form of vaginismus or dyspareunia.[26,28] This is thought to be due to a combination of lack of knowledge and pervasive social attitudes that tend to discount the importance of women's sexual functioning. One study from Lebanon surveyed gynecologists regarding their practice in screening for sexual dysfunction. A significant proportion indicated that they did not screen for sexual dysfunction or complaints, and half indicated that they had not had sufficient training.[29]

Men, on the other hand, are frequently reported to suffer from sexual dysfunction secondary to performance anxiety. Some men with erectile dysfunction (ED) may feel that this is a result of witchcraft. They may seek advice from traditional healers.[30] One study reported that approximately 80% of men presenting to the physician with ED had previously consulted traditional healers.[26]

There are very few studies that report the prevalence of STDs in the region. One study suggested that presumed STDs were not uncommon in one rural population,[31] while others have reported a low prevalence of such infections.[32-7] Available evidence from small studies suggests that risk factors for STDs are similar to those in other parts of the world.[32,38-42] Overall, STDs are reported to be uncommon in the Arab world, primarily due to strong religious and cultural imperatives that discourage extramarital sexual contact.[43] While these cultural factors represent a strong defense against the propagation of STDs within the community, the proscribed nature of the subject also inhibits educational efforts and population surveillance.[44] One study that reviewed known human immuno-deficiency virus (HIV) cases among Arabs living in Israel reported that although the rate of infection was one-third that of the general population, they experienced a significantly longer delay between contracting the infection and detection.[42]

With exposure to the media, rapid cultural change, social and political instability, and increased mobility, people in the Arab world may be at higher risk for STDs in the future. In an unpublished study that surveyed students from four universities in Egypt, 25% of all male and 3% of female students reported having had sexual intercourse at least once.[45] Surveys from Lebanon are reported to show similar results.[46]

Close-kin marriage

Consanguineous marriage is defined by clinical geneticists as being a union between second cousins or closer relations. In Arab countries, the rate of consanguineous marriages has been reported to range between 20% and 70%.[47,48] It has been postulated that this nuptial pattern meets a number of family and individual needs. These include:

- consolidating family wealth and property
- ensuring spouses for their own children by reciprocation
- minimizing individual and family stress by encouraging the couple to remain close to kin
- taking advantage of pre-existing support and coalition patterns in the family.

The social preference for unions between close relatives is seen in many parts of the world, including southern India, Latin America, South Africa and Japan. The practice of close-kin marriage is sanctioned by a number of religions, including Judaism, Buddhism and the Zoroastian/Parsis. The position of Islam on close-kin marriage is more ambiguous.[49] However, close-kin marriage was reportedly common in pre-Islamic Arab society.[50] This may account for its presence among members of all faiths in the region.[51,52]

Several studies have established that the children of parents who were first cousins were significantly more likely to marry close relatives than the offspring of less closely related parents.[13,53,54] This is concordant with studies from other parts of the world that report strong correlations between parents' consanguinity and that of their children.

Although the highest rates of consanguineous marriages have traditionally been reported to occur in rural areas and areas where there are lower levels of education,[55-7] the data are not consistent; other studies report no significant educational differences between individuals in consanguineous and non-consanguineous marriages.[58-60] Some studies seem to indicate that consanguinity, particularly first cousin marriage, is correlated with high educational attainment among the husbands in these marriages[54,56,61] and discordance in spousal education.[62] Some authorities have speculated that since an educated man becomes a more valuable asset, additional effort is made to keep him close to the family.[56] It is tempting to consider education as an isolated factor mediating the rate of consanguineous marriage within families. However, the preponderance of the available data seem to indicate that the extent of family and community involvement in facilitating marriage arrangements is the factor most responsible for the prevalence of consanguinity in a given community.

From a family dynamics perspective, in a close-knit collective community, higher education may represent a kind of "moving away" from the family in a symbolic and sometimes a literal sense. In this context, added encouragement to take a close relative in marriage represents a reciprocal shift of family "toward" the one who is moving "away".

It is reported that genetic disorders in Arab countries account for a considerable proportion of disease burden due to mental and physical disabilities.[63,64] Much of this genetic disease burden is thought to derive from high consanguinity rates in the region (*see also* Chapter 4, Genetic disorders). Several studies from the Levant and the Gulf reviewing pregnancy outcomes of consanguineous unions report that they do not suffer from an increased incidence of prematurity, abortion or low birth weight. However, they do result in significantly higher neonatal mortality and congenital malformations.[55,65-9] A study that explored risk factors for abortion among women living in rural Egypt reported consanguinity as a significant factor. Although the incidence of induced abortion was not likely to be high in this population, the study did not differentiate between induced and spontaneous abortions.[70]

One study noted increased severity of reading disability among the offspring of more closely related parents in a group of Arab students with learning disabilities who resided in Israel.[71]

Several studies report that there is widespread awareness of the potential genetic consequences of close-kin marriage among members of both consanguineous and non-consanguineous marriages.[72,73] Although some studies report that consanguineous marriage is less common among Christians than Muslims, there appears to be no difference in awareness of the potential genetic consequences between the two groups.[58]

The social imperative that influences marital patterns is very strong; it is not unusual for closely related couples to proceed with marriage arrangements and have children despite the knowledge that they are at very high risk of having a child with a specific genetic disorder.[74] Furthermore, couples who already have offspring affected by genetic disorders frequently continue to favor consanguineous unions for themselves and their children.[75]

At times, the family motivation encouraging consanguineous marriages may be less than benign, and coercion or deception may occur. One study of 150 individuals in discordant marriages presenting to an outpatient psychiatric clinic in Saudi Arabia found that consanguineously married individuals were more likely to have met each other briefly or not at all before marriage. Of this group, significant numbers suffered from a psychotic disorder such as schizophrenia, an anxiety disorder, or dysthymic disorder.[76] In some cases, families may encourage disabled members to marry close kin in order to ensure a spouse and ongoing care for the disabled individual.

There is some evidence to indicate that women in particular may experience psychosocial and health benefits from being in a consanguineous union. It has been proposed that close-kin marriage may be socially advantageous for women by allowing them to take advantage of pre-existing support and alliances within the family.[77] A report from Syria suggested that women in consanguineous unions were less likely to be smokers.[78]

One study reported that women who were married to relatives had better relationships with their in-laws than did controls.[73] Another study found that women who were in non-cousin marriages were more likely to suffer from psychiatric morbidity than those who were married to relatives.[79] These findings contradict the results of a smaller study of low income women in Syria that did not detect a significant correlation between close-kin marriage and psychiatric morbidity.[80] Given the high rates of psychiatric morbidity in the sample, however, it is unclear whether the study had sufficient statistical power to demonstrate a difference between the groups.

Polygamous marriage

In the Arab world, polygamous marriage is defined as a marital relationship involving more than one wife. There are no accurate statistics on the prevalence of polygamy in the general population among Muslims in the Arab world. Authorities indicate that trends in the prevalence of polygamy change over time, and vary by region,[81] although it is generally accepted to be much less prevalent than was formerly the case.[82] Polygamy seems to be more common in Muslim communities that adhere closely to traditional lifestyles. However, there is little in-depth research about this family arrangement, apart from some studies of polygamy and polygamous families among the Bedouin living in the Negev. Therefore, this section will review the available literature with this caveat in mind.

In Muslim communities, polygamous marriage offers an alternative to divorce or widowhood in a society where a previously married woman and her children's prospects may be bleak. Historically, this marriage arrangement has also served protective, restorative and remedial functions in communities decimated by warfare.[83]

Islam permits polygamous marriage of up to four wives only if sufficient economic resources are available, and all wives and families receive equal attention, resources and treatment. However, a review of the available literature suggests that these ideals are frequently disregarded. Instead, the sanction allowing multiple marriage may be exploited to satisfy personal desires, or to punish or retaliate against a wife and/or her family. Frequently, a second marriage will be sought if there are problems with infertility, mental illness or incompatibility.[84] Additionally, in some groups it is hypothesized that women who consent to enter into a polygamous union (usually second wives) tend to be less socially desirable,[85] and therefore may have higher rates of pre-existing physical, psychiatric or behavioral disorders. These potentially confounding factors should be investigated in future studies.

Research has documented a number of associations between polygamous marital structure and health and health behavior, primarily among women. One study from Egypt reported that polygamously married women were more likely to reject postpartum medroxyprogesterone acetate contraceptive injections than women in monogamous unions. This was presumably due to "fertility competitiveness" between wives.[86] Conversely, a study from Morocco reported that women in polygamous unions were more likely to use contraception.[87] Reports from Kuwait, the United Arab Emirates (UAE), Jordan, Syria, Palestine and Israel have described involvement in a polygamous marriage as a significant risk factor for mental health problems in women, including anxiety, depression and somatization.[79,80,84,88–91] A polygamous family structure was also identified as a risk factor for mental health and academic problems in children and adolescents among Bedouins in the Negev[92] and the UAE,[93] however, a later study of a pediatric primary care population in the UAE found no significant association between polygamy and psychiatric morbidity.[94] Some authors have noted a scenario in which much older men marry additional wives and sire children, but do not survive long enough to raise them, leaving the wives and children with emotional, social and economic difficulties.[95]

More nuanced studies have suggested that the negative psychosocial impact of polygamy is more strongly linked to the specifics of the individual marital relationship and community attitudes than it is to the specific nuptial arrangement.[76,96,97] Slonim-Nevo and Al-Krenawi, in a qualitative study that compared well-functioning and poorly functioning polygamous families with two wives among the Bedouin of the Negev desert, suggested that factors leading to successful adjustment to a polygamous marriage included:

- the decision to take a second wife was shared with the first wife before the marriage, and the first wife was supported and involved throughout the process
- the first wife felt that the circumstances leading to the marriage outweighed her own desires and interests
- both wives and families were treated equally
- the households were maintained separately
- wives respected each others' roles, and were able to settle disagreements amicably.[97]

In summary, women in polygamous unions appear to be at risk for certain health conditions, related to the psychosocial issues surrounding this arrangement. Personal, family and community factors are likely to play a major role in whether or not polygamy is a risk factor for these conditions. A truly objective assessment of whether or not polygamous marriage arrangements are disproportionately harmful should compare the effects of alternative marital outcomes (such as divorce) to this arrangement.

Divorce

Broken marriages have many implications for marriage partners, their families and society at large.[98–100] Divorce has also been shown to have a considerable impact on the mental health and economic well-being of families and individuals.[101] Cross-national studies suggest that reasons for divorce, the divorce process and outcomes of divorce are strongly modulated by cultural factors.[102–5] Little literature exists that explores divorce and its impacts on individuals and families in the Arab world. What is available, however, may provide a starting point for understanding the dynamics and effects of divorce in Arab countries, and generating hypotheses for further investigations.

One study explored the reasons given for divorce by 312 Muslim men and women living in Israel. Although problems of communication and incompatibility were cited by a majority of both sexes, physical abuse, substance abuse, interference by family members and infertility were commonly mentioned as causes for divorce. Men were more likely to mention infertility problems, while more women cited physical abuse.[106]

Studies confirm the general impression that divorce has a disproportionate impact on women in the social, psychological and economic arenas. One study that explored predictors of better adjustment after divorce found that these factors included being male, being employed and having a good education. It also reported that women suffered from more mental distress than men due to issues surrounding the divorce.[107]

A major consequence of divorce for women is the severe social stigma that accompanies this state. Studies report that women experience diminished social status, increased dependence on their family of origin, limitations of social and economic opportunities and increases in family discord.[107–10] This can result in enormous stress. Several studies have reported that divorced women exhibit very high rates of somatic and psychological symptoms.[79,108,111] Another interesting finding is that, in contrast to the literature from other parts of the world, the number of years since divorce does not predict better adjustment to the post-divorce state among women.[107] This suggests that the social stigma attached to divorced women in Arab populations is persistent and probably permanent.[112,113]

Reproductive health

Reproductive health has been defined by the World Health Organization as "a state of physical, mental and social well being in all matters relating to the reproductive system at all stages of life".[114] Implicit in this definition are the abilities to experience a safe and satisfying sexual life, have access to appropriate healthcare services for pregnancy and childbirth, and have access to measures to control fertility if desired.[115]

Addressing reproductive health is a highly cost-effective way to reduce disease burden and simultaneously address larger social development needs. Measures that improve reproductive health are often intimately linked to many health and development issues such as women's education, reductions in childhood mortality, and promotion of environmental sustainability through population control. The reproductive health infrastructure also provides a convenient "point of first contact" for many individuals and their families within the larger healthcare system.

Although there have been major improvements in the healthcare of women in the Arab world in the past few decades as measured by maternal and perinatal morbidity and mortality, significant inequities continue to plague both access to services and overall health status among women. These inequities are primarily related to region, education and income, and represent barriers to the provision of consistently high-quality reproductive healthcare in the region.

Reproductive, maternal and perinatal morbidity/mortality

Among women of reproductive age, complications of pregnancy and childbirth are leading causes of illness and death. This is particularly true in developing countries. Maternal mortality remains a leading cause of illness and death of women in their reproductive years in a number of Arab countries,[116] while in other areas, rates approach those of developed European nations.

A number of factors are thought to have contributed to the uneven progress of improvement in maternal and perinatal mortality rates in many Arab countries. Factors such as political instability and the growing prevalence of chronic diseases may deplete government resources that might otherwise be utilized for maternal and perinatal care. Other factors include absence of planning and policy guidelines for reproductive health, poor quality of available services, and lack of development of other critical sectors. Cultural and social barriers may also play a role.[117]

Biologically, the process of childbearing in humans is demanding and perilous. Most maternal deaths occur around the time of delivery, or shortly thereafter. Therefore, the biggest reductions in maternal mortality can be attained by providing all pregnant women with high-quality delivery care and adequate back-up and referral systems in case of emergency. Further important reductions can be attained by the provision of good quality prenatal and postnatal care. An emerging concept is the provision of "preconception care" as a complement to antenatal care. Preconception care is defined as the provision of medical and behavioral interventions prior to conception that improve subsequent health and pregnancy outcomes.[118] This might include premarital screening for genetic conditions such as thalassemia, counseling regarding adequate nutrient intake, vaccination, and the detection and treatment of infections.

However, optimal reductions in maternal mortality rates are not due solely to directly applied medical resources. Maternal health is also closely dependent on more global aspects of good community, individual, physical and psychosocial health. These include: community awareness regarding health issues that include pregnancy and childcare, education and literacy, as well as contraceptive and birthspacing options. This is illustrated by the fact that women who begin having children at an early age, women who have frequent, closely spaced pregnancies, and those who suffer from anemia or chronic infections such as tuberculosis or malaria, are much more likely to die in childbirth.

A fundamental requirement for individuals to seek healthcare is to perceive that a health problem exists. A ground-breaking study from rural Egypt found that the single most important factor affecting women's utilization of healthcare services was the perception of their own health status.[119] Particularly in rural and poorly literate populations, women are seldom able to detect a serious health problem that might require medical care. This highlights the critical role that women's education plays in improving the quality of reproductive healthcare. Similar studies in other countries suggest a high prevalence of unaddressed reproductive health problems among women,[120–5] particularly urinary tract infections, genital prolapse and non-specific vaginitis.

One study from Jordan demonstrated that a brief community-based educational intervention had a significant effect on health awareness among rural-dwelling women.[126] Social, cultural and environmental barriers are also important in the decision to seek care for health issues.[122] Several studies reported that while reproductive problems were common among women in rural Egypt, women rarely sought medical care for, or discussed, these problems with others.[127] One study of women living in rural Egypt found that one-quarter of women who had experienced a miscarriage reported having been afraid to tell their husband of symptoms, such as vaginal bleeding, that they had experienced prior to the event.[70]

Barriers to obtaining healthcare include:
- poor education (no perception of a health problem)
- cultural barriers (e.g. a preference for seeking help from traditional healers, or the unavailability of female health providers)
- geographic barriers (no nearby health facility)
- socioeconomic barriers (no money to pay for care)
- organizational barriers (e.g. long wait times for an appointment, or no wheelchair access).

Fertility and contraception

Motherhood and successful childbearing are the dominant features in the self-image of many women, and may be the only roles open to them in the societies in which they live. Therefore, successful childbearing is often the only avenue to a woman's social, emotional and economic fulfilment. Social preferences and pressures may result in frequent, closely spaced pregnancies in the quest for an "acceptable" number of children of the "correct" gender.[128,129]

This sociocultural dynamic translates into the early marriage and childbearing seen in many regions where a traditional lifestyle is the norm. In this setting, women who delay marriage are often at risk for loss of social worth and marriageability. Those who delay childbearing after marriage often face pressure from the extended family to prove their fecundity. While the value of delayed marriage, educational attainment and the recognition of women's potential outside the domestic setting is gradually becoming more valued in many parts of the Arab world, these recent attitudes seem to be linked to urbanization, education and increased incomes. In general, women from lower socioeconomic and rural populations are much more likely to adhere to traditional patterns of marriage and childbearing.

A report from Syria suggested that in urban areas, the wife's educational level has the strongest impact on family size, while in rural areas, the husband's education correlates more strongly with smaller family size.[130]

Given the strong cultural pressure on both men and women to adhere to traditional norms, it is not surprising that contraception and limiting childbearing are seen by many as a mixed blessing, despite the economic benefits that might accrue from having fewer children.

Although historically the Arab world was considered an homogeneous area in which high fertility was persistent, some researchers assert that, in fact, patterns of fertility decline in the Arab world are similar to those seen in other parts of the developing world after the introduction of effective programs for birth control and birthspacing.[131] These declines are thought to have been largely due to the development of explicit family planning policies and improved access to reproductive healthcare. However, there is evidence that declines in fertility may also be due to other factors. In a number of countries, fertility declines due to adverse economic conditions have been observed.[132,133] It is also hypothesized that complex social forces that include improved education among both men and women, and gradual transformation of the economic environment, are driving the ongoing fertility declines that are being observed.[134]

Although the declines in fertility rates have been promising, significant numbers of families continue to have unmet needs for family planning (families who desire to control their fertility but are unable to do so).[135] Unmet needs for birth control are most acute among rural dwellers and those from lower socioeconomic populations. Reasons for unmet need include inaccessible or poor-quality reproductive health services, where women may not be adequately educated on birth control methods, may receive inappropriate methods, or may not be offered birth control at all. One barrier for many women is the absence of female providers trained in reproductive healthcare. These healthcare barriers often result in high rates of contraceptive non-use or discontinuation, and subsequent undesired fertility.[136,137]

Many studies have been carried out that explore women's use of contraception. Factors that have been reported to affect the use of contraception among couples are summarized below.

Reported risk factors for contraceptive non-use among couples:[129,138,139, 140,141–51,156]

- early marriage
- family pressure to have children
- no male offspring
- illiteracy or low educational attainment
- being rural dwellers
- personal or religious beliefs of the woman, her husband or family
- lack of access to health facilities with female providers.

One study from the UAE found that, contrary to other studies from Arab countries, women in higher socioeconomic groups were actually less likely to be users of contraception.[148] Similarly, a study of adolescents' attitudes toward contraception in Oman revealed that individuals were less likely to expect people from upper socioeconomic classes to use contraception.[23]

Making high-quality, accessible reproductive healthcare available to women is one way to increase contraceptive uptake in a population. Another is to consider any contact with the healthcare system an opportunity for women to receive information about or obtain contraception. Also important but often neglected is the role that others, such as friends and family members, play in a woman's decision to use contraception. Involvement of the husband in making the decision to use contraception has been noted in several studies.[139,143,147,152–4] One study from Egypt found that integrating contraceptive education into routine antenatal visits and involving the husband in these visits increased contraceptive use after delivery.[155] A Cochrane review also found that postpartum contraceptive education was effective in increasing rates of contraceptive use.[156] Patients who were engaged collaboratively by their physicians in the clinical encounter at which they received contraceptive advice were more likely to be continuing use of the method at their seven-month follow-up.[157] Innovative methods, such as the insertion of intrauterine contraceptive devices (IUDs) immediately postpartum, have also found to be effective in increasing rates of contraceptive uptake.[158]

Community level interventions in many countries have built on strong cultural norms that encourage good health among all family members. Introducing the concept of "birthspacing" – or planned births that are spaced optimally to allow for recovery of the mother's health between pregnancies, adequate attention to each child, and the economic benefits that flow from having smaller families, has shown promise.

Religion and contraception

A number of studies have explored the role of religion, specifically Islam, and its relationship to contraceptive utilization in the Arab world.[139,142,143,159–61] The preponderance of the evidence suggests that while the attitudes and practices of the populations studied are diverse, most seem to agree with the liberal interpretations of Islamic scholars on matters of birth control.[162] In fact, studies

---

1991 Judgments regarding contraception by the Grand Imam of Al-Azhar[166]

■ Contraception (by whatever means) is permissible.

■ Permanent sterilization should be performed only to safeguard the health of the mother.

■ Induced abortion after 120 days of gestation is forbidden except to save the mother's life. (Prior to this time, it is permitted only if certified that the fetus has a serious untreatable condition.)

---

suggest that the factors having the strongest effect on contraceptive utilization are perceptions of contraceptive efficacy, safety and availability.[163] One study from Yemen reported that the strongest correlate of visit regularity to a family planning clinic was the availability of high-quality services; religion seemed to play a less significant role.[164] This assessment is strengthened by a study from India that found no difference in the rate of contraception adoption between Hindu and Muslim populations of the same socioeconomic status.[165]

However, some studies have noted that among subjects who were non-users of contraception, the perception that religious teaching forbids contraception was common.[148,149,151]

Forms of contraception

Studies from throughout the Arab world show consistency in the types of contraception used by women. In interpreting many of these studies, however, it should be noted that these findings often apply primarily to women of middle to low income groups who are the subjects of many of these studies. The most common practice reported is "coitus interruptus" or withdrawal of the penis before ejaculation. The rhythm method is reportedly widely used. These methods have the advantage of having unanimous religious and social sanction, and are cost free, but they are only moderately effective. The introduction of the lactational amenorrhea method of birth control (LAM) is a promising one for increasing birth intervals. This method requires that new mothers nurse their babies on demand, and switch to a back-up birth control method if menses occur. The advantages of this method are that it promotes breastfeeding and is cost free. Disadvantages include the intensiveness of breastfeeding required; this makes LAM particularly difficult for working women to utilize.

Among modern contraceptive methods, the most popular is the intrauterine device (IUD). This has the advantages of being effective and requiring little ongoing maintenance, but may be associated with pain, bleeding and infection. Further, placement of the device requires a trained operator, preferably a female, for maximal acceptability. Placement of the device immediately postpartum may overcome some of the barriers to its use. Oral contraceptive tablets are also utilized, and it has been reported that this method is more popular among people in higher socioeconomic groups.[167] It has been reported that "skewing" of contraceptive method use occurs in many countries[168] because patients are pressured overtly or covertly toward a particular method. This may be due to availability and cost of the method rather than to true preference.[169]

Condoms are used infrequently. One study from Lebanon reported that poor spousal communication and a lingering sense of social stigma are some causes of non-use.[170] A report from the UAE found that men described various perceived unpleasant consequences of condom use, such as discomfort and reduced sexual pleasure.[149] In a study involving Jordanian men, unfavorable attitudes toward condom use were also reported.[143]

The role of misinformation and rumors may also be important in the uptake of contraceptive methods by a population.[171,172]

Studies from other regions of the world demonstrate that personal experience and accounts from social networks are often more powerful in shaping peoples' perceptions of contraceptive safety than medical opinion.[173]

TABLE 3.1 Commonly used contraceptive methods

TYPE	DESCRIPTION	ADVANTAGES	DISADVANTAGES
coitus interruptus	withdrawal prior to ejaculation	traditional method; well accepted; no side-effects	high failure rate
rhythm method (safe period)	intercourse only during times of the month when fertilization and implantation are least likely	no cost; universally sanctioned; no side-effects	only moderately effective in usual practice (failure rate 25% per year); only reliable if ovulation and menses regular
condoms	barrier method may be used with spermicide to increase efficacy	low cost; few or no side-effects; prevents transmission of sexually transmitted diseases (STDs)	inconsistent use due to embarrassment, poor communication and perception of reduced sensation
diaphragm	barrier method inserted over the cervix, used with a spermicide	few or no side-effects; good efficacy; reduced STD transmission	requires fitting by medical professional; needs to be inserted by user prior to each intercourse; frequently not well accepted by conservative individuals
lactational amenorrhea method (LAM)	breastfeeding of newborn on demand results in high prolactin levels leading to ongoing anovulation and amenorrhea	effective and has health benefits for mother and baby; no side-effects; no cost	intensive breastfeeding schedule may be difficult for some individuals; can only be used reliably for six months postpartum
intrauterine contraceptive device (IUD, IUCD)	device inserted into the uterus where it maintains hostile environment for implantation	effective; no-systemic side effects; no action needed after insertion; lasts several years	need for a trained operator to insert; requires pelvic exam; leads to increased incidence of menstrual cramping, bleeding, risk of infection

cont.

TYPE	DESCRIPTION	ADVANTAGES	DISADVANTAGES
medroxyprogesterone acetate injection (Depo-Provera)	progestogenic agent maintains anovulatory state	lasts three months; given by intramuscular injection; effective	recommended to be used no longer than two years; risk of osteoporosis; hormonal side-effects (weight gain, headache etc.); may cause irregular menstrual bleeding
oral contraceptive pills	estrogens and progestogens induce anovulation	effective; generally well tolerated; can be used over the long term	hormonal side-effects; needs to be taken daily; increased risk of stroke in smokers and older women

Infertility

A number of studies have explored the effects of infertility on women in Arab countries. Given the social and cultural imperative for a married couple to have children, infertility places women at risk for social stigmatization and rejection. Some authors report that, in some populations, women who have borne many children and who experience reduced fertility due to age may present to the physician for fertility evaluation if it is feared that the husband might marry another wife.[174] Studies report that many infertile women experience high levels of psychiatric distress, and even suicidal ideation,[175] particularly among women in polygamous marriages.[176] Frequently, infertile women seek care from traditional healers, or other unscrupulous practitioners. It has been reported that with some women who are married to infertile partners, there is an expectation to acknowledge publicly that the infertility is the wife's fault rather than their husband's, to save him from undue embarrassment.[177]

Healthcare providers should be aware of the high levels of social and psychiatric risk that infertile women face, and should thoroughly evaluate and provide support for these women.

Female genital cutting

The term "female genital cutting" (FGC) refers to a number of related traditional cultural practices found in various parts of the world, including Africa, Australia and parts of Indonesia and the Philippines. FGC has been defined as amputation of any part of the female genitalia for non-medical purposes. In the Arab world, FGC is reported to be widespread in Somalia, Sudan[178] and Egypt. Reports also reference the practice of FGC among some populations in a number of other countries such as Jordan,[179] Saudi Arabia[180] and Oman.[23] FGC may be performed on girls in infancy, childhood or adolescence, but is usually performed between four and 12 years of age. FGC is reported to occur among members of all faith groups, including Muslims, Christians, Jews and Animists.[181]

Among the groups who practice it, FGC is seen as a critical part of a woman's cultural identity. A woman who does not undergo the procedure may be seen as unclean, unmarriageable and prone to unethical sexual behavior by members of her community. This places a great deal of social pressure on the family to comply with tradition.

In 1995 the World Health Organization classified FGC procedures into four broad descriptive categories:[182]

➡ *type I:* excision of the clitoral hood with or without removal of the clitoris

➡ *type II:* removal of the clitoris together with part or all of the labia minora

(Types I and II account for about 85% of cases.)

➡ *type III (infibulation):* removal of part or all of the external genitalia including clitoris as well as labia majora and minora, then stitching the remaining introitus leaving a small opening for urine and menstrual flow

➡ *type IV (unclassified):* all other operations on the female genitalia, including piercing, or incision of the clitoris and/or labia; cauterization by burning the clitoris and genital tissues; incisions of the vaginal wall, and other procedures.

Many medical groups and international organizations have condemned the practice of FGC, classifying it as a violation of human rights since it is performed without informed consent. It also may result in severe consequences including infection, chronic pain, disability and obstetric morbidity.[183] Others advocate a more conservative approach, arguing that there is little objective evidence that these procedures cause significant harm,[184] and pointing to male circumcision as being an analogous genital procedure that is routinely performed without informed consent. Governmental efforts to eliminate the practice, some of which have dated back to the 1920s,[185] have been largely unsuccessful.[186] However, it has been noted in recent years that attitudes among women toward FGC are changing; younger women are much less likely to look upon FGC favorably than were women from previous generations.[45]

Health screening and disease prevention

The objective of health screening is to reduce morbidity and mortality rates of a specified disease or diseases in a defined population, in a cost-effective manner. In order for a program of screening to accomplish these objectives, the following criteria must be met:

➡ the disease must present a significant *health burden* in the population in question

➡ the disease should have a significant period during which it is *asymptomatic,* so that early detection and treatment will yield improvement in the medical outcome

➡ the screening test or tests must be *acceptable* to the population screened, as well as being *safe, sensitive and specific*; the *costs* of screening should be reasonable.

It can be seen from the criteria set out above that what constitutes a reasonable screening program can vary a great deal from one country to another depending on prevalence of disease, availability of resources and community acceptance factors. For example, studies that have explored the feasibility of screening programs for cervical cancer have discovered many obstacles to implementation of programs. One study from the UAE suggested that the combination of a low prevalence of cervical cancer and a conservative population who might find screening unacceptable might not be cost-efficient.[187] Other studies suggest that factors such as the lack of training of medical personnel,[188] and fear and embarrassment on the part of patients, represent significant barriers to implementation of this type of screening.[189]

The concept of periodic screening for occult illness is a relatively new one for many. This is often true for both providers and consumers of medical care, as the perceived need for this type of illness prevention is relatively recent. To many providers, health screening may represent an added burden to their traditional duties, and they may not have received appropriate training[188] or resources to fulfill screening requirements. Additionally, the traditional healthcare "disease treatment" model is not an arrangement that is easily modified to include the elements needed to incorporate prevention and screening into day-to-day care. A shift from curative to preventive healthcare delivery is a profound one, and requires changes to the entire structure of the healthcare system, and not just at the clinic level.[190]

A number of studies have explored attitudes, behaviors and barriers to women's health prevention and screening in the Arab world. One study from Jordan reported that although women performed well on some aspects of health promotion, they scored poorly in taking responsibility for their own health.[191] Some authors have highlighted women's difficulty in accessing healthcare generally due to family and community pressures. Other barriers are reported to include lack of knowledge about screening, and preference for female health providers due to issues of embarrassment and modesty.[192]

Example: Breast cancer screening

Breast cancer is a major health problem for women worldwide. It is the most common cause of female cancer and female cancer deaths in both developing and developed areas of the world.[193] Although breast cancer cannot be prevented, a number of risk factors for the disease have been noted. Among these are age, reproductive history, family history of breast cancer, dietary factors and environmental exposures.

Currently, secondary prevention of breast cancer is the only method that will reliably reduce morbidity and mortality from this disease. Secondary prevention is accomplished through early detection and treatment of breast cancer. Three modalities – clinical breast examination (CBE), breast self-examination (BSE) and mammography – are commonly used for screening. These tests allow earlier identification of tumors, earlier treatment and improved outcomes. Unfortunately, simply making services available for screening is not enough to ensure that people will take advantage of them. One theoretical framework, known as the Health Belief Model (*see also* Chapter 17, Patient education), may serve to illustrate the dynamics associated with health behavior, particularly behavior related to health screening.

The Health Belief Model

Factors increasing the likelihood that an individual will take action to deal with a health related issue include:

- a perception that one is personally susceptible to a health problem or condition
- a perception that the problem is harmful, and the magnitude of the harmfulness
- an interest in preserving or improving one's personal health
- a perception that taking a particular action (in this case, screening) will have benefits
- a perception that barriers to taking action (seeking screening) do not exist.

In Arab countries, a number of barriers exist in the implementation of breast cancer screening programs. One frequently encountered issue is the lack of funding for education and screening programs. Several studies have highlighted the fact that women suffer from a lack of knowledge about breast cancer; this is in part due to sporadic health education about breast cancer by medical personnel.[194,195] One study highlighted the low expectations that some health providers had regarding the benefit of educating patients.[196] Another found that women received less health education than did men in a diabetes clinic.[197] A qualitative study from the UAE identified the existence of factors that both encouraged and deterred breast cancer screening among Emerati women.[198]

Although a lack of knowledge among women about breast cancer was a dominant theme in the studies, several other psychosocial factors seemed to play an important role. The first was denial. This fundamental psychological defense mechanism prevents overwhelming anxiety in a variety of settings. Denial can interfere with appropriate planning and action if it is persistent. This cognitive pattern is seen among people of all educational levels and national origins. Denial, together with a prevailing cultural belief in predestination or "fate", may be a particularly powerful combination of factors that discourage women from seeking screening.

Another issue reported to be important is the stigma associated with having a potentially deadly condition. In a society with a strongly collective ethos, individuals are socialized to maintain their assigned roles; one's sense of connection and life purpose is often closely linked to the role that one is assigned by society. A diagnosis of cancer threatens a woman's role as mother and caregiver. Therefore, cancer may be seen not only as a life-threatening condition but also as a potential threat to her status as a family and community member. Similar findings have been reported among ethnic Chinese women living in Australia,[199,200] and Puerto Rican and Dominican women living in the United States.[201]

TABLE 3.2 Encouraging and discouraging factors in breast cancer screening among women[194,195,198,202-4]

Encouraging factors
- feelings of susceptibility or vulnerability to cancer
- experience of a first-degree relative with breast cancer
- support from family and community
- belief in personal responsibility for health
- belief in God's will acting through the medical personnel
- knowledge about breast cancer, screening and outcomes
- trust in the healthcare system
- recommendation of screening by health personnel
- lack of barriers to screening.

Discouraging factors
- misconceptions and low knowledge about breast cancer and medical outcomes
- embarrassment and modesty
- fear of pain with screening
- belief in supernatural causation of illness and in faith healing
- belief that fate prevails over personal responsibility for health
- fear of loss of role and subsequent community rejection
- lack of recommendation for screening by healthcare personnel.

Women and mental health

Poor mental health is a major health burden for women worldwide. Women make up about 70% of the people who seek mental healthcare in most countries. Recently it has been hypothesized that the observed excess mental illness seen in women may be an artifact based on cultural roles and pressures; these lead men to exhibit psychological distress preferentially through substance abuse and violence, while women are encouraged to express, or "internalize" this discomfort through depression and anxiety.

Internationally, women are more likely to suffer from poor education, poverty and discrimination than are men.[205] Therefore, much psychological distress in women is a result of their relative vulnerability to adverse life experiences, expectations and attitudes.

In the Arab world, although community surveys have confirmed that women are more likely to suffer from psychiatric illness than men, a number of studies report that more men than women seek mental health services,[27,206] although one study from the UAE reported equal rates of mental health utilization.[207] This is thought to be partly due to the severe stigma associated with mental illness,[208] and the willingness of relatives to care for people who are highly disabled within the family.[209] Women may also preferentially experience and express their symptoms as "nerves", "fatigue" or other idioms of distress that may not be understood by health professionals.[210] Somatization, or the expression of physical symptoms to convey psychological distress, is another common scenario that draws attention away from the true cause of the distress in the clinical setting.

Many studies from the Arab world describe the impact that social issues have on women's mental health. Issues such as occupational stress,[211] marital strife, separation and divorce,[79,111,212] as well as family conflict,[80] all have profound impacts on women's psychosocial well-being. Women who are in dysfunctional family relationships are also more likely to suffer from postpartum depression.[89,213] Anxiety, which tends to be more prevalent in women internationally, is common among girls and women in the Arab world.[93,214–16] Anxiety is also frequently co-morbid with depression, and chronic anxiety often leads to major depression over time.

These findings echo studies from the West, which demonstrate, for example, that women in unhappy marriages have a 25-fold higher risk of depression than those in happy marriages.[217] Research that explores many aspects of women's mental health and the effects of culture change on mental health still needs to be done in the Arab world.

Other health issues

Partly as a consequence of the priorities of non-governmental and other organizations operating in the region, much of the focus on women's health research has involved matters related to reproduction. However, many other aspects of women's health differ significantly from those of men. These include susceptibility to and the course of conditions as varied as heart disease and osteoporosis. Both biological and social factors are thought to be responsible for these differences. Very little research has been carried out thus far in the Arab world on these conditions. It is hoped that in the future, researchers will focus their attention on some of these issues.

References

1 Kickbusch I. Health promotion: key public health strategy for the MENA/EM region. In: Pierre-Louis A, Akala F, Karam H, editors. *Public Health in the Middle East and North Africa: meeting the challenges of the twenty-first century.* Washington, DC: The World Bank; 2004, p. 71.

2 Shawki S, Milaat W, Abalkhalil B *et al.* Effect of maternal education on the rate of childhood handicap. *Saudi Medical Journal* 2001; **22 (1):** 39–43.

3 Eapen V, Zoubeidi T, Yunis F *et al.* Prevalence and psychosocial correlates of global developmental delay in 3-year-old children in the United Arab Emirates. *J Psychosom Res* 2006; **61 (3):** 321–6.

4 Anon. Gender and citizenship initiative. In: *United Nations Development Programme,* Geneva, 2004.

5 Al-Qutob R, Mawajdeh S, Allosh R *et al.* The effect of prenatal knowledge of fetal sex on birth weight: a study from Jordan. *Health Care Women Int* 2004; **25 (3):** 281–91.

6 El-Gilani A, Shady E. Determinants and causes of son preference among women delivering in Mansoura, Egypt. *Eastern Mediterranean Health Journal* 2007; **13 (1):** 119–28.

7 Kamel HS, Ahmed HN, Eissa MA *et al.* Psychological and obstetrical responses of mothers following antenatal fetal sex identification. *J Obstet Gynaecol Res* 1999; **25 (1):** 43–50.

8 Abdelmoneim I. A study of determinants of low birth weight in Abha, Saudi Arabia. *Afr J Med Sci* 2004; **33 (2):** 145–8.

9 Maziak W, Mzayek F, al-Musharref M. Effects of environmental tobacco smoke on the health of children in the Syrian Arab Republic. *East Mediterr Health J* 1999; **5 (4):** 690–7.

10 Ahmed FA. Gender difference in child mortality. *Egypt Popul Fam Plann Rev* 1990; **24 (2):** 60–79.

11 Obermeyer CM, Cardenas R. Son preference and differential treatment in Morocco and Tunisia. *Stud Fam Plann* 1997; **28 (3):** 235–44.

12 Arnold F. *Gender Preferences for Children.* Demographic and Health Surveys, Comparative Studies number 23. Claverton, MD: Macro International; 1997.

13 Klat M, Khudr A. Religious endogamy and consanguinity in marriage patterns in Beirut, Lebanon. *Soc Biol* 1986; **33 (1–2):** 138–45.

14 Abou Shabana K, el-Shiek M, el-Nazer M *et al.* Women's perceptions and practices regarding their rights to reproductive health. *East Mediterr Health J* 2003; **9 (3):** 296–308.

15 Schvaneveldt P, Kerpelman J, Schvaneveldt J. Generational and cultural changes in family life in the United Arab Emirates: a comparison of mothers and daughters. *Journal of Comparative Family Studies* 2005; **36 (1):** 77–91.

16 Bint Ahmad Jaffer Y, Afifi M. Adolescents' attitudes toward gender roles and women's empowerment in Oman. *East Mediterr Health J* 2005; **11 (4):** 805–18.

17 Lev-Weisel R, Al-Krenawi A. Attitude toward marriage and marital quality: a comparison among Israeli Arabs differentiated by religion. *Family Relations* 1999; **48 (1):** 51–6.

18 El-Islam M. Mental illness in Kuwait and Qatar. In: Al-Issa I, editor. *Al-Junun: mental illness in the Muslim world.* Madison, CT: International Universities Press Inc.; 2000. pp. 127–8.

19 Al-Issa I. Culture and mental illness in Algeria. In: Al-Issa I, editor. *Al-Junun: mental illness in the Islamic world.* Madison, CT: International Universities Press Inc.; 2000. pp. 116–17.

20 Bayer R, Shunaigat W. Psychological, social and cultural aspects of unconsummated marriage. *Arab Journal of Psychiatry* 2001; **12 (2):** 43–52.

21 Al-Sughayir M. Unconsummated marriage: a Saudi version. *Arab Journal of Psychiatry* 2004; **15 (2):** 122–30.

22 Bedri NM. Grandmothers' influence on mother and child health. *Ahfad J* 1995; **12 (1):** 74–86.

23 Jaffer YA, Afifi M, Al Ajmi F *et al.* Knowledge, attitudes and practices of secondary-school pupils in Oman: II. Reproductive health. *East Mediterr Health J* 2006; **12 (1–2):** 50–60.

24 De Jong J, Shepherd B, Mortagy I *et al. The Reproductive Health of Young People in the Middle East and North Africa.* Presented at IUSSP Conference in Tours, France; July 2005.

25 Shakhatreh F, Odibat A. *Assessment of Health and Social Needs of Females in the Age Group 9–65 Years in South Jordan.* Amman, Jordan: University of Jordan; 2003.

26 Al-Sawaf M, Al-Issa I. Sex and sexual dysfunction in an Arab-Islamic society. In: Al-Issa I, editor. *Al-Junun: mental illness in the Islamic world.* Madison, CT: International Universities Press Inc.; 2000. pp. 295–311.

27 Douki S, Nacef F. Women's mental health in Tunisia. *World Psychiatry* 2002; **1 (1):** 55–6.

28 Chaleby K, Jabbar J, Al-Sawaf M. Psychotherapy of sexual dysfunction in Arab patients. *Arab Journal of Psychiatry* 1996; **7 (2):** 99–110.

29 El-Kak F, Jurdi R, Kaddour A *et al.* Gender and sexual health in clinical practice in Lebanon. *Int J Gynaecol Obstet* 2004; **87 (3):** 260–6.

30 Alsugharyir M. Public view of the "evil eye" and its role in psychiatry. *Arab Journal of Psychiatry* 1996; **7 (2):** 152–60.

31 Al-Qutob R, Mawajdeh S, Massad D. Can a home-based pelvic examination be used in assessing reproductive morbidity in population-based studies? A Jordanian experience. *J Adv Nurs* 2001; **33 (5):** 603–12.

32 Al-Qutob, Mawajdeh S, Khateeb M *et al.* The magnitude of reproductive tract infections/Sexually transmitted infections in selected sites in Jordan. In: Medical Islamic Conference; 2004; Amman, Jordan; 2004.

33 Deeb M, Ghorayeb F, Kabakian-Khasholian T *et al.* Measuring gynecological morbidity: evaluating two different data sources from Beirut. *Health Care Women Int* 2003; **24 (3):** 254–65.

34 El-Sayed NM, Gomatos PJ, Rodier GR *et al.* Seroprevalence survey of Egyptian tourism workers for hepatitis B virus, hepatitis C virus, human immunodeficiency virus, and *Treponema pallidum* infections: association of hepatitis C virus infections with specific regions of Egypt. *Am J Trop Med Hyg* 1996; **55 (2):** 179–84.

35 Malkawi SR, Abu Hazeem RM, Hajjat BM *et al.* Evaluation of cervical smears at King Hussein Medical Centre, Jordan, over three and a half years. *East Mediterr Health J* 2004; **10 (4–5):** 676–9.

36 Ibrahim AI, Kouwatli KM, Obeid MT. Frequency of herpes simplex virus in Syria based on type-specific serological assay. *Saudi Med J* 2000; **21 (4):** 355–60.

37 Madani TA. Sexually transmitted infections in Saudi Arabia. *BMC Infect Dis* 2006; **6:** 3.

38 Mostafa SR, Roshdy OH. Risk profiles for sexually transmitted diseases among patients attending the venereal disease clinic at Alexandria Main University Hospital. *East Mediterr Health J* 1999; **5 (4):** 740–54.

39 Adib SM, Akoum S, El-Assaad S *et al.* Heterosexual awareness and practices among Lebanese male conscripts. *East Mediterr Health J* 2002; **8 (6):** 765–75.

40 Ismail SO, Ahmed HJ, Grillner L *et al.* Sexually transmitted diseases in men in Mogadishu, Somalia. *Int J STD AIDS* 1990; **1 (2):** 102–6.

41 Madani TA, Al-Mazrou YY, Al-Jeffri MH *et al.* Epidemiology of the human immunodeficiency virus in Saudi Arabia; 18-year surveillance results and prevention from an Islamic perspective. *BMC Infect Dis* 2004; **4: 25.**

42 Chemtob D, Srour SF. Epidemiology of HIV infection among Israeli Arabs. *Public Health* 2005; **119 (2):** 138–43.

43 Lenton C. Will Egypt escape the AIDS epidemic? *Lancet* 1997; **349 (9057):** 1005.

44 De Jong J, Jawad R, Mortagy I *et al.* The sexual and reproductive health of young people in the Arab countries and Iran. *Reprod Health Matters* 2005; 13 (25): 49–59.

45 Khalil T, Boog J, Salem R. *Addressing the Reproductive Health Needs and Rights of Young People since ICPD: the contribution of UNFPA and IPPF.* University of Heidelberg; 2003.

46 Al-Kak F. *Background Paper on Reproductive and Sexual Health in the Eastern Mediterranean Region.* Beirut: American University of Beirut; 2003.

47 Hoodfar E, Teebi AS. Genetic referrals of Middle Eastern origin in a western city: inbreeding and disease profile. *J Med Genet* 1996; **33 (3):** 212–15.

48 Teebi AS, El-Shanti HI. Consanguinity: implications for practice, research, and policy. *Lancet* 2006; **367 (9515):** 970–1.

49 Bittles A. Consanguinity and its relevance to clinical genetics. *Clin Genet* 2001; **60 (2):** 89–98.

50 Rajab A, Patton MA. A study of consanguinity in the Sultanate of Oman. *Ann Hum Biol* 2000; **27 (3):** 321–6.

51 Vardi-Saliternik R, Friedlander Y, Cohen T. Consanguinity in a population sample of Israeli Muslim Arabs, Christian Arabs and Druze. *Ann Hum Biol* 2002; **29 (4):** 422–31.

52 Cohen T, Vardi-Saliternik R, Friedlander Y. Consanguinity, intracommunity and intercommunity marriages in a population sample of Israeli Jews. *Ann Hum Biol* 2004; **31 (1):** 38–48.

53 Hamamy H, Jamhawi L, Al-Darawsheh J *et al.* Consanguineous marriages in Jordan: why is the rate changing with time? *Clin Genet* 2005; **67 (6):** 511–16.

54 Bener A, Abdulrazzaq YM, al-Gazali LI *et al.* Consanguinity and associated socio-demographic factors in the United Arab Emirates. *Hum Hered* 1996; **46 (5):** 256–64.

55 Al Husain M, Al Bunyan M. Consanguineous marriages in a Saudi population and the effect of inbreeding on prenatal and postnatal mortality. *Ann Trop Paediatr* 1997; **17 (2):** 155–60.

56 Khoury SA, Massad D. Consanguineous marriage in Jordan. *Am J Med Genet* 1992; **43 (5):** 769–75.

57 Eshra DK, Dorgham LS, el-Sherbini AF. Knowledge and attitudes towards premarital counselling and examination. *J Egypt Public Health Assoc* 1989; **64 (1–2):** 1–15.

58 Jaber L, Shohat M, Halpern GJ. Demographic characteristics of the Israeli Arab community in connection with consanguinity. *Isr J Med Sci* 1996; **32 (12):** 1286–9.

59 Al-Salem M, Rawashdeh N. Consanguinity in north Jordan: prevalence and pattern. *J Biosoc Sci* 1993; **25 (4):** 553–6.

60 Kerkeni E, Monastiri K, Saket B *et al.* Association among education level, occupation status, and consanguinity in Tunisia and Croatia. *Croat Med J* 2006; **47 (4):** 656–61.

61 Jurdi R, Saxena PC. The prevalence and correlates of consanguineous marriages in Yemen: similarities and contrasts with other Arab countries. *J Biosoc Sci* 2003; **35 (1):** 1–13.

62 Al-Kandari Y, Crews DE, Poirier FE. Consanguinity and spousal concordance in Kuwait. *Coll Antropol* 2002; **26 Suppl:** 1–13.

63 Al-Gazali L, Hamamy H, Al-Arrayad S. Genetic disorders in the Arab world. *BMJ* 2006; **333 (7573):** 831–4.

64 Barbari A, Stephan A, Masri M *et al.* Consanguinity-associated kidney diseases in Lebanon: an epidemiological study. *Mol Immunol* 2003; **39 (17–18):** 1109–14.

65 Bromiker R, Glam-Baruch M, Gofin R *et al.* Association of parental consanguinity with congenital malformations among Arab newborns in Jerusalem. *Clin Genet* 2004; **66 (1):** 63–6.

66 Khoury SA, Massad DF. Consanguinity, fertility, reproductive wastage, infant mortality and congenital malformations in Jordan. *Saudi Med J* 2000; **21 (2):** 150–4.

67 Al-Gazali LI, Bener A, Abdulrazzaq YM *et al.* Consanguineous marriages in the United Arab Emirates. *J Biosoc Sci* 1997; **29 (4):** 491–7.

68 Al-Hosani HA, Brebner J, Bener AB *et al.* Study of mortality risk factors for children under age 5 in Abu Dhabi. *East Mediterr Health J* 2003; **9 (3):** 333–43.

69 Abdulrazzaq YM, Bener A, al-Gazali LI *et al.* A study of possible deleterious effects of consanguinity. *Clin Genet* 1997; **51 (3):** 167–73.

70 Yassin KM. Incidence and socioeconomic determinants of abortion in rural Upper Egypt. *Public Health* 2000; **114 (4):** 269–72.

71 Abu-Rabia S, Maroun L. The effect of consanguineous marriage on reading disability in the Arab community. *Dyslexia* 2005; **11 (1):** 1–21.

72 Jaber L, Romano O, Halpern GJ *et al.* Awareness about problems associated with consanguineous marriages: survey among Israeli Arab adolescents. *J Adolesc Health* 2005; **36 (6):** 530.

73 Khlat M, Halabi S, Khudr A *et al.* Perception of consanguineous marriages and their genetic effects among a sample of couples from Beirut. *Am J Med Genet* 1986; **25 (2):** 299–306.

74 Raz A, Atar M. Upright generations of the future: tradition and medicalization in community genetics. *Journal of Contemporary Ethnography* 2004; **33 (3):** 296–322.

75 Al-Gazali LI. Attitudes toward genetic counseling in the United Arab Emirates. *Community Genet* 2005; **8 (1):** 48–51.

76 Chaleby K. Traditional Arabian marriages and mental health in a group of outpatient Saudis. *Acta Psychiatr Scand* 1988; **77 (2):** 139–42.

77 Yanca C, Low B. Female allies and female power: a cross cultural analysis. *Evolution and Human Behavior* 2004; **25 (1):** 9–23.

78 Maziak W, Asfar T, Mzayek F. Socio-demographic determinants of smoking among low-income women in Aleppo, Syria. *Int J Tuberc Lung Dis* 2001; **5 (4):** 307–12.

79 Daradkeh T, Alawan A, Al-Ma'aitah R *et al.* Psychiatric morbidity and its sociodemographic correlates among women in Irbid, Jordan. *Eastern Mediterranean Health Journal* 2006; **12 (Suppl 2):** S-107-17.

80 Maziak W, Asfar T, Mzayek F *et al.* Socio-demographic correlates of psychiatric morbidity among low-income women in Aleppo, Syria. *Soc Sci Med* 2002; **54 (9):** 1419–27.

81 Chamie J, Weller RH. Levels, trends and differentials in nuptiality in the Middle East and North Africa. *Genus* 1983; **39 (1–4):** 213–31.

82 Prothro ET, Diab LN. *Changing Family Patterns in the Arab East.* Beirut: American University of Beirut; 1974.

83 Khaliq U. Beyond the veil: an analysis of the provisions of the women's convention in the law as stipulated in the Shari'a. *Buffalo Journal of International Law* 1995; **2:** 1–47.

84 Chaleby K. Women of polygamous marriages in an inpatient psychiatric service in Kuwait. *J Nerv Ment Dis* 1985; **173 (1):** 56–8.

85 Johnson NE, Elmi AM. Polygamy and fertility in Somalia. *J Biosoc Sci* 1989; **21 (2):** 127–34.

86 Younis MN, Nadeem Ne-M, Salem HI *et al.* Factors affecting acceptability of long-acting contraceptive injections in a rural Egyptian community. *J Biosoc Sci* 1987; **19 (3):** 305–11.

87 Varea C, Crognier E, Bley D *et al.* Determinants of contraceptive use in Morocco: stopping behaviour in traditional populations. *J Biosoc Sci* 1996; **28 (1):** 1–13.

88 Al-Krenawi A, Graham J, Izzeldin A. The psychosocial impact of polygamous marriages on Palestinian women. *Women and Health* 2001; **34 (1):** 1–16.

89 Abou-Saleh MT, Ghubash R. The prevalence of early postpartum psychiatric morbidity in Dubai: a transcultural perspective. *Acta Psychiatr Scand* 1997; **95 (5):** 428–32.

90 Al-Krenawi A, Graham JR. A comparison of family functioning, life and marital satisfaction, and mental health of women in polygamous and monogamous marriages. *Int J Soc Psychiatry* 2006; **52 (1):** 5–17.

91 Nasir LS, Al-Qutob R. Barriers to the diagnosis and treatment of depression in Jordan: a nationwide qualitative study. *J Am Board Fam Pract* 2005; **18 (2):** 125–31.

92 Al-Krenawi A, Lightman ES. Learning achievement, social adjustment, and family conflict among Bedouin-Arab children from polygamous and monogamous families. *J Soc Psychol* 2000; **140 (3):** 345–55.

93 Eapen V, Al-Gazali L, Bin-Othman S *et al.* Mental health problems among schoolchildren in United Arab Emirates: prevalence and risk factors. *J Am Acad Child Adolesc Psychiatry* 1998; **37 (8):** 880–6.

94 Eapen V, Al-Sabosy M, Saeed M *et al.* Child psychiatric disorders in a primary care Arab population. *Int J Psychiatry Med* 2004; **34 (1):** 51–60.

95 Fakhr El-Islam M. Mental illness in Kuwait and Qatar. In: Al-Issa I, editor. *Al-Junun: Mental Illness in the Islamic World.* Madison, CT: International Universities Press, Inc.; 2000. p. 131.

96 Al-Krenawi A, Graham JR, Slonim-Nevo V. Mental health aspects of Arab-Israeli adolescents from polygamous versus monogamous families. *J Soc Psychol* 2002; **142 (4):** 446–60.

97 Slonim-Nevo V, Al-Krenawi A. Success and failure among polygamous families: the experience of wives, husbands, and children. *Fam Process* 2006; **45 (3):** 311–30.

98 Huurre T, Junkkari H, Aro H. Long-term psychosocial effects of parental divorce: a follow-up study from adolescence to adulthood. *Eur Arch Psychiatry Clin Neurosci* 2006; **256 (4):** 256–63.

99 Isir AB, Tokdemir M, Kucuker H *et al.* Role of family factors in adolescent delinquency in an Elazig/Turkey reformatory. *J Forensic Sci* 2007; **52 (1):** 125–7.

100 Nock SL. Marriage as a public issue. *Future Child* 2005; **15 (2):** 13–32.

101 Anda RF, Brown DW, Felitti VJ *et al.* Adverse childhood experiences and prescribed psychotropic medications in adults. *Am J Prev Med* 2007; **32 (5):** 389–94.

102 Goode WJ. *World Changes in Divorce Patterns.* New Haven: Yale University Press; 1993.

103 Kitson GC, Babri KB, Roach MJ. Who divorces and why: a review. *J Fam Issues* 1985; **6 (3):** 255–93.

104 Kidd MP. The impact of legislation on divorce: a hazard function approach. *Appl Econ* 1995; **27 (1):** 125–30.

105 Neyrand G, M'Sili M. Mixed couples in contemporary France: marriage, acquisition of French nationality and divorce. *Popul* 1998; **10 (2):** 385–416.

106 Cohen O, Savaya R. Reasons for divorce among Muslim Arabs in Israel: an exploratory study. *European Societies* 2003; **5 (3):** 303–25.

107 Cohen O, Savaya R. Adjustment to divorce: a preliminary study among Muslim Arab citizens of Israel. *Fam Process* 2003; **42 (2):** 269–90.

108 Al-Krenawi A. Somatization among Bedouin-Arab women differentiated by marital status. *Journal of Divorce and Remarriage* 2004; **42 (1–2):** 131–43.

109 Cohen O, Savaya R. "Broken Glass": the divorced woman in Moslem Arab society in Israel. *Fam Process* 1997; **36 (3):** 225–45.

110 Al-Krenawi A. Divorce among Muslim Arab women in Israel. *Journal of Divorce and Remarriage* 1988; **29 (3–4):** 103–19.

111 Hamid H, Abu-Hijleh NS, Sharif SL *et al.* A primary care study of the correlates of depressive symptoms among Jordanian women. *Transcult Psychiatry* 2004; **41 (4):** 487–96.

112 Savaya R, Cohen O. Perceptions of the societal image of Muslim Arab divorced men and women in Israel. *Journal of Social and Personal Relationships* 2003; **20 (2):** 193–202.

113 Darweesh K, Hadiah R, Atallah K *et al.* Effect of some variables on the status of divorced women: an exploratory study on a sample of divorcees in Amman. *Dirasat* 1995; **22 A (Suppl):** 3301–21.

114 Raymond SU, Greenberg HM, Leeder SR. Beyond reproduction: women's health in today's developing world. *Int J Epidemiol* 2005; **34 (5):** 1144–8.

115 *Progress in Human Reproduction Research* Number 45. 1998 [cited 2007, 15 May]. Available from: www.who.int/reproductive-health/hrp/progress/45/prog45.pdf.

116 Mahaini R, Mahmoud H. Maternal health in the eastern Mediterranean region of the World Health Organization. *East Mediterr Health J* 2005; **11 (4):** 532–8.

117 Aoyama A. *Reproductive Health in the Middle East and North Africa*. Washington, DC: The International Bank for Reconstruction and Development; 2001, p. xxi.

118 Agrey N, Crowe K, Levitt C *et al.* Preconception care. In: Hanvey L, editor. *Family Centered Maternal and Newborn Care: national guidelines.* Ottawa: Health Canada, Ministry of Public Works and Services; 2005, p. 3.1–3.29.

119 Khattab HAS, Younis N, Zurayk H *et al. Women, Reproduction, and Health in Rural Egypt: the Giza study.* Cairo, Egypt: American University in Cairo Press; 1999.

120 Mawajdeh SM, Al-Qutob R, Schmidt A. Measuring reproductive morbidity: a community-based approach, Jordan. *Health Care Women Int* 2003; **24 (7):** 635–49.

121 Al-Qutob R. Menopause-associated problems: types and magnitude: a study in the Ain Al-Basha area, Jordan. *J Adv Nurs* 2001; **33 (5):** 613–20.

122 Al-Qutob R, Majali S, Massad D *et al.* Perceptions of health and seeking care: the experience of midlife women in Ain Al-Basha, Jordan. *The International Quarterly of Community Health Education* 1999–2000; **19 (2):** 163–78.

123 Deeb ME, Awwad J, Yeretzian JS *et al.* Prevalence of reproductive tract infections, genital prolapse, and obesity in a rural community in Lebanon. *Bull World Health Organ* 2003; **81 (9):** 639–45.

124 Rizk DE, Shaheen H, Thomas L *et al.* The prevalence and determinants of health care-seeking behavior for urinary incontinence in United Arab Emirates women. *Int Urogynecol J Pelvic Floor Dysfunct* 1999; **10 (3):** 160–5.

125 [In Egypt, researchers assess the health of village women.] *Safe Mother* 1991 **(6):** 3.

126 Schmidt A, Al-Qutob R, Mawajdeh S *et al.* Raising women's reproductive health awareness: a community-based intervention program in Jordan. *Annals of Saudi Medicine* 2003; **23 (1–2):** 76–80.

127 Rural Egyptian women bear heavy disease burden. *Popul Briefs* 2000; **6 (2):** 5.

128 Khalaf I, Callister LC. Cultural meanings of childbirth: Muslim women living in Jordan. *J Holist Nurs* 1997; 15 (4): 373–88.

129 Gadalla S, McCarthy J, Campbell O. How the number of living sons influences contraceptive use in Menoufia Governorate, Egypt. *Stud Fam Plann* 1985; **16 (3):** 164–9.

130 Alloush K. Fertility preferences and contraceptive use. In: Farid S, Alloush K, editors. *Reproductive Patterns in Syria.* Voorburg, Netherlands: International Statistical Institute; 1987.

131 Rashad H. Demographic transition in Arab countries: a new perspective. *Population Research* 2000; **17 (1):** 83–101.

132 Fargues P. State policies and the birth rate in Egypt: from socialism to liberalism. *Population and Development Review* 1997; **23 (1):** 115–38.

133 Courbage Y. [The Arabian Peninsula: demographic surprises.] *Maghreb Machrek* 1994; **144:** 3–25.

134 Fargues P. Women in Arab countries: challenging the patriarchal system? *Reprod Health Matters* 2005; **13 (25):** 43–8.

135 Casterline JB, El-Zanatay F, El-Zeini LO. Unmet need and unintended fertility: longitudinal evidence from upper Egypt. *Int Fam Plan Perspect* 2003; **29 (4):** 158–66.

136 Al-Qutob R, Mawajdeh S, Nawar L *et al. Assessing the Quality of Reproductive Health Services.* Giza, Egypt: The Population Council Regional Office for West Asia and North Africa; 1998.

137 Mawajdeh S, Family Health Group, Primary Health Team. *Unmet Needs and Missed Opportunities for Family Planning Among Married Women 15–49 Years Users of MOH Health Centers: Primary Health Care Initiatives (PHCI)*; November 2004. Report No.: MAARD No. OUTNMS 106. Initiatives Inc.

138 Sallam SA, Mahfouz AA, Dabbous NI. Reproductive health of married adolescent women in squatter areas in Alexandria, Egypt. *East Mediterr Health J* 2001; 7 **(6):** 935–42.

139 Kridli SA, Libbus K. Contraception in Jordan: a cultural and religious perspective. *Int Nurs Rev* 2001; **48 (3):** 144–51.

140 Chebaro R, El Tayyara L, Ghazzawi F *et al.* [Knowledge, attitudes and practices about contraception in an urban population.] *East Mediterr Health J* 2005; **11 (4):** 573–85.

141 Youssef RM. Duration and determinants of interbirth interval: community-based survey of women in southern Jordan. *East Mediterr Health J* 2005; **11 (4):** 559–72.

142 Libbus K, Kridli S. Contraceptive decision making in a sample of Jordanian Muslim women: delineating salient beliefs. *Health Care Women Int* 1997; **18 (1):** 85–94.

143 Petro-Nustas W, Al-Qutob R. Jordanian men's attitudes and views of birth-spacing and contraceptive use (a qualitative approach). *Health Care Women Int* 2002; **23 (6–7):** 516–29.

144 Youssef RM, Moubarak, II, Gaffar YA *et al.* Correlates of unintended pregnancy in Beheira governorate, Egypt. *East Mediterr Health J* 2002; 8 **(4–5):** 521–36.

145 Ali MM. Quality of care and contraceptive pill discontinuation in rural Egypt. *J Biosoc Sci* 2001; **33 (2):** 161–72.

146 Yount KM, Langsten R, Hill K. The effect of gender preference on contraceptive use and fertility in rural Egypt. *Stud Fam Plann* 2000; **31 (4):** 290–300.

147 Abu Ahmed A, Tabenkin H, Steinmetz D. [Knowledge and attitudes among women in the Arab village regarding contraception and family planning and the reasons for having numerous children.] *Harefuah* 2003; **142 (12):** 822–5, 878, 879.

148 Ghazal-Aswad S, Rizk DE, Al-Khoori SM *et al.* Knowledge and practice of contraception in United Arab Emirates women. *J Fam Plann Reprod Health Care* 2001; **27 (4):** 212–16.

149 Ghazal-Aswad S, Zaib-Un-Nisa S, Rizk DE *et al.* A study on the knowledge and practice of contraception among men in the United Arab Emirates. *J Fam Plann Reprod Health Care* 2002; **28 (4):** 196–200.

150 Farid S. Fertility and family planning in the Arab region. *IPPF Med Bull* 1986; **20 (1):** 1–3.

151 Saghayroun AA, Khalifa MA. Fertility and Islam in the Sudan. *Sudan J Popul Stud* 1984; **1 (2):** 1–28.

152 Khalifa MA. Attitudes of urban Sudanese men toward family planning. *Stud Fam Plann* 1988; **19 (4):** 236–43.

153 Warren CW, Hiyari F, Wingo PA *et al.* Fertility and family planning in Jordan: results from the 1985 Jordan Husbands' Fertility Survey. *Stud Fam Plann* 1990; **21 (1):** 33–9.

154 El-Zanaty FH. Women segmentation based on contraceptive use. *Egypt Popul Fam Plann Rev* 1994; **28 (1):** 19–54.

155 Soliman MH. Impact of antenatal counselling on couples' knowledge and practice of contraception in Mansoura, Egypt. *East Mediterr Health J* 1999; **5 (5):** 1002–13.

156 Hiller J. Education for contraceptive use by women after childbirth. In: *Cochrane Database Syst Rev;* 2002.

157 Abdel-Tawab N, Roter D. The relevance of client-centered communication to family planning settings in developing countries: lessons from the Egyptian experience. *Soc Sci Med* 2002; **54 (9):** 1357–68.

158 Grimes D, Schulz K, van Vliet H *et al.* Immediate post-partum insertion of intrauterine devices: a Cochrane review. *Hum Reprod* 2002; **17 (3):** 549–54.

159 Sabbah I, Drouby N, Sabbah S *et al.* Quality of life in rural and urban populations in Lebanon using SF-36 Health Survey. *Health Qual Life Outcomes* 2003; **1 (1):** 30.

160 Sueyoshi S, Al-Khozahe HO, Ohtsuka R. Effects of reproduction norms on contraception practice among Muslim women in Amman, Jordan. *Eur J Contracept Reprod Health Care* 2006; **11 (2):** 138–45.

161 Sueyoshi S, Ohtsuka R. Ineffective contraceptive use and its causes in a natural fertility population in southern Jordan. *Hum Biol* 2004; **76 (5):** 711–22.

162 Bignall J. Family planning in Islam (Abstract). *Lancet* 1993; **341 (8846):** 687.

163 Albsoul-Younes AM, Saleh F, El-Khateeb W. Perception of efficacy and safety as determinants for use and discontinuation of birth control methods in Muslim Jordanian women. *Eur J Contracept Reprod Health Care* 2003; **8 (3):** 156–61.

164 Inaoka E, Wakai S, Nakamura Y *et al.* Correlates of visit regularity among family planning clients in urban Yemen. *Adv Contracept* 1999; **15 (4):** 257–74.

165 Iyer S. Religion and the decision to use contraception in India. *Journal for the Scientific Study of Religion* 2002; **41 (4):** 711–22.

166 Omran AR. *Family Planning in the Legacy of Islam.* London; New York: Routledge; 1992.

167 Al-Gallaf K, al-Wazzan H, al-Namash H *et al.* Ethnic differences in contraceptive use in Kuwait: a clinic-based study. *Soc Sci Med* 1995; **41 (7):** 1023–31.

168 Sullivan TM, Bertrand JT, Rice J *et al.* Skewed contraceptive method mix: why it happens, why it matters. *J Biosoc Sci* 2006; **38 (4):** 501–21.

169 *Quality of Family Planning Services.* 1994 [cited 2006, 11 December]. Available from: http://www.unfpa.org/monitoring/pdf/n-issue3.pdf

170 Kulczycki A. The sociocultural context of condom use within marriage in rural Lebanon. *Stud Fam Plann* 2004; **35 (4):** 246–60.

171 Family planning dialogue. Rumors of contraception: myths vs facts. *New Egypt J Med* 1990; **4 (2 Suppl):** 1–21.

172 DeClerque J, Tsui AO, Abul-Ata MF *et al.* Rumor, misinformation and oral contraceptive use in Egypt. *Soc Sci Med* 1986; **23 (1):** 83–92.

173 Guendelman S, Denny C, Mauldon J *et al.* Perceptions of hormonal contraceptive safety and side effects among low-income Latina and non-Latina women. *Matern Child Health J* 2000; **4 (4):** 233–9.

174 Shah NM, Shah MA, Radovanovic Z. Patterns of desired fertility and contraceptive use in Kuwait. *International Family Planning Perspectives* 1998; **24 (3):** 133–8.

175 Fido A. Emotional distress in infertile women in Kuwait. *Int J Fertil Women's Med* 2004; **49 (1):** 24–8.

176 Khayata GM, Rizk DE, Hasan MY *et al.* Factors influencing the quality of life of infertile women in United Arab Emirates. *Int J Gynaecol Obstet* 2003; **80 (2):** 183–8.

177 Inhorn MC. Middle Eastern masculinities in the age of new reproductive technologies: male infertility and stigma in Egypt and Lebanon. *Med Anthropol Q* 2004; **18 (2):** 162–82.

178 Satti A, Elmusharaf S, Bedri H *et al.* Prevalence and determinants of the practice of genital mutilation of girls in Khartoum, Sudan. *Ann Trop Paediatr* 2006; **26 (4):** 303–10.

179 Nasir S. *Study on Women's Health in Jordan.* Department of Sociology, University of Jordan, Amman, Jordan; 1996.

180 Abu Daia JM. Female circumcision. *Saudi Med J* 2000; **21 (10):** 921–3.

181 Gilbert D. For the sake of purity (and control). Female genital mutilation. *Links* 1993; **9 (5):** 6–8, 30.

182 Elmusharaf S, Elhadi N, Almroth L. Reliability of self reported form of female genital mutilation and WHO classification: cross sectional study. *BMJ* 2006; **333 (7559):** 124.

183 Banks E, Meirik O, Farley T *et al.* Female genital mutilation and obstetric outcome: WHO collaborative prospective study in six African countries. *Lancet* 2006; **367 (9525):** 1835–41.

184 Obermeyer CM. The consequences of female circumcision for health and sexuality: an update on the evidence. *Cult Health Sex* 2005; **7 (5):** 443–61.

185 Elchalal U, Ben Ami B, Brzezinski A. Female circumcision: the peril remains. In: Whitfield H, editor. *Circumcision Supplement.* Oxford: British Journal of Urology; 1999.

186 Magoha GA, Magoha OB. Current global status of female genital mutilation: a review. *East Afr Med J* 2000; **77 (5):** 268–72.

187 Ghazal-Aswad S, Gargash H, Badrinath P *et al.* Cervical smear abnormalities in the United Arab Emirates: a pilot study in the Arabian Gulf. *Acta Cytol* 2006; **50 (1):** 41–7.

188 Badrinath P, Ghazal-Aswad S, Osman N *et al.* A study of knowledge, attitude, and practice of cervical screening among female primary care physicians in the United Arab Emirates. *Health Care Women Int* 2004; **25 (7):** 663–70.

189 Bakheit N, Bu Haroon A. The knowledge, attitude and practice of Pap smear among local school teachers in the Sharjah district. *Middle East Journal of Family Medicine* 2004; **4 (4).**

190 Ferguson RS. Preventive care in daily practice. *J Okla State Med Assoc* 2000; **93 (4):** 154–60.

191 Al Ma'aitah R, Haddad L, Umlauf MG. Health promotion behaviors of Jordanian women. *Health Care Women Int* 1999; **20 (6):** 533–46.

192 Rizk DE, El-Zubeir MA, Al-Dhaheri AM *et al.* Determinants of women's choice of their obstetrician and gynecologist provider in the UAE. *Acta Obstet Gynecol Scand* 2005; **84 (1):** 48–53.

193 Bray F, McCarron P, Parkin DM. The changing global patterns of female breast cancer incidence and mortality. *Breast Cancer Res* 2004; **6 (6):** 229–39.

194 Petro-Nustus W, Mikhail BI. Factors associated with breast self-examination among Jordanian women. *Public Health Nurs* 2002; **19 (4):** 263–71.

195 Cohen M, Azaiza F. Early breast cancer detection practices, health beliefs, and cancer worries in Jewish and Arab women. *Prev Med* 2005; **41 (5–6):** 852–8.

196 Haddad LG, Umlauf MG. Views of health promotion among primary health care nurses and midwives in Jordan. *Health Care Women Int* 1998; **19 (6):** 515–28.

197 Abdelmoneim I, Al-Homrany MA. Health education in the management of diabetes at the primary health care level: is there a gender difference? *East Mediterr Health J* 2002; **8 (1):** 18–23.

198 Bener A, Alwash R, Miller CJ *et al.* Knowledge, attitudes, and practices related to breast cancer screening: a survey of Arabic women. *J Cancer Educ* 2001; **16 (4):** 215–20.

199 Kwok C, Sullivan G. Influence of traditional Chinese beliefs on cancer screening behaviour among Chinese-Australian women. *J Adv Nurs* 2006; **54 (6):** 691–9.

200 Kwok C, Sullivan G. Chinese-Australian women's beliefs about cancer: implications for health promotion. *Cancer Nurs* 2006; **29 (5):** E14–21.

201 Goldman RE, Risica PM. Perceptions of breast and cervical cancer risk and screening among Dominicans and Puerto Ricans in Rhode Island. *Ethn Dis* 2004; **14 (1):** 32–42.

202 Baron-Epel O, Granot M, Badarna S *et al.* Perceptions of breast cancer among Arab Israeli women. *Women Health* 2004; **40 (2):** 101–16.

203 Azaiza F, Cohen M. Health beliefs and rates of breast cancer screening among Arab women. *J Women's Health* 2006; **15 (5):** 520–30.

204 Bener A, Honein G, Carter AO *et al.* The determinants of breast cancer screening behavior: a focus group study of women in the United Arab Emirates. *Oncol Nurs Forum* 2002; **29 (9):** E91–8.

205 Stewart DE, Rondon M, Damiani G *et al.* International psychosocial and systemic issues in women's mental health. *Archives of Women's Mental Health* 2001; **4:** 13–17.

206 Al-Subaie A, Marwa M, Hawari R *et al.* Psychiatric emergencies in a university hospital in Riyadh, Saudi Arabia. *International Journal of Mental Health* 1997; **4 (25):** 59–68.

207 Daradkeh TK, Ghubash R, Abou-Saleh MT. Al Ain Community Survey of Psychiatric Morbidity III. The natural history of psychopathology and the utilization rate of psychiatric services in Al Ain. *Soc Psychiatry Psychiatr Epidemiol* 2000; **35 (12):** 548–53.

208 El-Islam MF, Abu-Dagga S. Marriage and fertility rates of schizophrenic patients in Kuwait. *Med Principles Pract* 1990; **2:** 18–26.

209 El-Islam MF. Rehabilitation of schizophrenics by the extended family. *Acta Psychiatr Scand* 1982; **65 (2):** 112–19.

210 McIlvenny S, DeGlume A, Elewa M *et al.* Factors associated with fatigue in a family medicine clinic in the United Arab Emirates. *Fam Pract* 2000; **17 (5):** 408–13.

211 Hattar-Pollara M, Meleis AI, Nagib H. Multiple role stress and patterns of coping of Egyptian women in clerical jobs. *J Transcult Nurs* 2003; **14 (2):** 125–33.

212 Khatwa SA, Abdou MH. Adult depression in Alexandria, Egypt, 1998. *J Egypt Public Health Assoc* 1999; **74 (3–4):** 333–52.

213 Green K, Broome H, Mirabella J. Postnatal depression among mothers in the United Arab Emirates: socio-cultural and physical factors. *Psychol Health Med* 2006; **11 (4):** 425–31.

214 Abdel-Khalek AM, Lester D. Anxiety in Kuwaiti and American college students. *Psychol Rep* 2006; **99 (2):** 512–14.

215 Mikhail BI, Ragheb MS. Health-related concerns and experiences of employed perimenopausal women in Alexandria, Egypt. *Health Care Women Int* 1996; **17 (2):** 173–86.

216 Abou-Saleh MT, Ghubash R, Daradkeh TK. Al Ain Community Psychiatric Survey. I. Prevalence and socio-demographic correlates. *Soc Psychiatry Psychiatr Epidemiol* 2001; **36 (1):** 20–8.

217 Lundblad AM, Hansson K. Outcomes in couple therapy: reduced psychiatric symptoms and improved sense of coherence. *Nord J Psychiatry* 2005; **59 (5):** 374–80.

CHAPTER 4

Genetic disorders

(★ *Ghazi O Tadmouri*

Introduction

Until recently, infectious or environmental diseases and malnutrition-related disorders constituted the major cause of ill health and mortality in Arab populations. However, progress made in healthcare standards in many Arab countries has decreased the impact of these disorders. Improved understanding of the spectrum of heritable disease and better recognition of genetically transmitted conditions as major causes of morbidity and mortality are increasing awareness of the importance of these conditions in the region.[1]

Arab populations and diasporas in the world

Arab populations encompass a vast geographical region that extends from Iraq in the east to Morocco in the west. They occupy the whole of Mesopotamia, the Levant, the Arabian Gulf, North Africa, as well as some parts of East and West Africa. Arab populations are distributed throughout 23 different countries, namely: Algeria, Bahrain, Comoros, Djibouti, Egypt, Eritrea, Iraq, Jordan, Kuwait, Lebanon, Libya, Mauritania, Morocco, Oman, Palestine, Qatar, Saudi Arabia, Somalia, Sudan, Syria, Tunisia, United Arab Emirates (UAE) and Yemen. The total population of these countries is approximately 315 million.

Throughout history, Arab emigrants formed many diasporas in other continents of the world. The main countries of emigration are, in order of percentage: Yemen, Jordan, Lebanon, Egypt, Syria, Morocco, Algeria, Tunisia, Mauritania and Sudan. The main countries of immigration within the Arab world are those of the Gulf Cooperation Council and Libya, which host more than two million Arabs. Outside the Arab world, the largest Arab communities live in Europe and North America. Arabs in the United Kingdom, Europe and the United States total some 12 million people, many of whom are well established.[2]

Demographic characteristics of Arab populations

Arabs are a large and heterogeneous group that resulted from the admixture with many other populations throughout history. Certain cultural and geographic considerations markedly affect the prevalence and natural history of genetic diseases in the Arab world. Some of these characteristics include:

- the presence of *isolates* (e.g. Armenians, Bedouins, Druzes, Jews, Kurds, Nubians and others) who share common gene pools due to recurrent inbreeding
- marriage at a young age[3]
- high birth rates (16–43 births per 1000 people)
- high infant mortality rate (10–76 deaths per 1000 live births)[4]
- childbearing at older maternal ages, often until menopause
- the lack of public health measures directed toward control and prevention of congenital and genetically determined disorders[3]
- large family sizes (2–7 children born per woman)
- high rates of inbreeding or consanguineous marriage – often a traditional practice followed within the same tribe, village or social unit.

Consanguinity in Arab people

One of the most important factors contributing to the preponderance of genetic disorders in Arab populations is the deep-rooted norm of consanguineous marriages. The term "consanguineous marriage" is defined as marriage between relatives. Geneticists usually classify unions between biologically related persons who are second cousins or closer as consanguineous.

Overall, it is estimated that 40–50% of marriages in the Arab world are consanguineous (*see* Figure 4.1). The specific types of consanguineous marriage vary between and within countries. First cousin marriages are the most common consanguineous bonds in the Arab world. Estimates indicate that the prevalence of first cousin marriages is approximately 11.4% in Egypt, 21% in Bahrain, 29% in Iraq, 30% in Kuwait, 31% in Saudi Arabia, and 32% in Jordan.

Religious, cultural and historical factors are important in maintaining the practice of consanguineous marriage. Contrary to popular assumptions, Islam does not advocate or encourage consanguineous marriages. In fact, Arabs probably practiced consanguinity long before the introduction of Islam in the 7th century. The preference for consanguineous marriage is not restricted to Islamic Arab communities. In some Christian communities (e.g. Lebanon), consanguinity is also common.

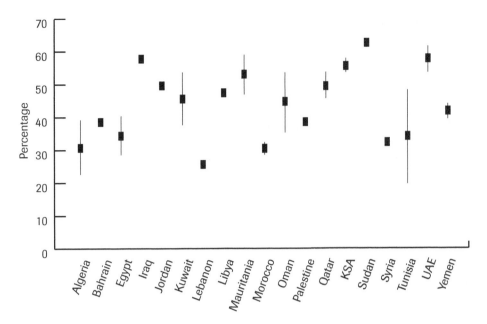

FIGURE 4.1 Percentage of consanguineous unions of total marriages in Arab countries Adapted from: Benallegue and Kedji, 1984 (Algeria);[5] ENAF, 1992 (Algeria);[6] Al-Arrayed, 1999 (Bahrain);[7] Hafez *et al.*, 1983 (Egypt);[8] ENPC, 1989 (Egypt);[9] Al-Hamamy *et al.*, 1986 (Iraq);[10] Khoury and Massad, 1992 (Jordan);[11] Al-Nasser *et al.*, 1989 (Kuwait);[12] Al-Awadi *et al.*, 1985 (Kuwait);[13] Klat and Khudr, 1986 (Lebanon);[14] Broadhead and Sehgal, 1981 (Libya);[15] National Statistical Office, 1992 (Mauritania);[16] Hammami *et al.*, 2005a (Mauritania);[17] Azelmat *et al.*, 1987 (Morocco);[18] Azelmat *et al.*, 1992 (Morocco);[19] Oman Family Health Survey, 1995 (Oman);[20] Rajab and Patton, 2000 (Oman);[21] Jaber *et al.*, 1992 (Palestine);[22] Ministry of Health, 1999 (Qatar);[23] Bener and Alali, 2006 (Qatar);[24] Wong and Anokute, 1990 (Saudi Arabia);[25] El-Hazmi *et al.*, 1995 (Saudi Arabia);[26] Saha *et al.*, 1990 (Sudan);[27] Prothro and Diab, 1974 (Syria);[28] Aloui *et al.*, 1988 (Tunisia);[29] Kerkeni *et al.*, 2006 (Tunisia);[30] Fahmy *et al.*, 1993 (UAE);[31] Al-Gazali *et al.*, 1995 (UAE);[32] Jurdi and Saxena, 2003 (Yemen);[33] Gunaid *et al.*, 2004 (Yemen).[34]

In addition to culture and history, the geographic concentration of population groups in small and isolated areas promoted the practice of consanguineous marriages. Many families also consider consanguineous marriage as a way to maintain the unity of family assets. Marriage to a relative is preferred, too, because of the comparative ease with which premarital negotiations can be conducted, and the greater stability of consanguineous unions due to familiarity between the female partner and her in-laws.[35]

Studies indicate that several factors influence consanguinity rates in Arabs. These factors include urban–rural residence ratios of families, education levels and time trends. Studies in Jordan,[11] Egypt, Lebanon, Oman and Tunisia demonstrated a higher tendency of consanguineous unions among rural compared to urban inhabitants.[33]

In some Arab countries, it is evident that the higher the level of education of the female partner, the lower the consanguinity rate.[11] On the contrary, in some societies, highly educated men are more likely to be married to cousins.[33] A plausible explanation is that since a son with higher education becomes a more valuable asset, he is pressured to remain within the family.[11]

While a declining trend of consanguineous marriages has been documented in Bahrain, Lebanon, Kuwait and Syria, a stable trend has been reported in Jordan and Oman.[33] However, these rates have increased over the last generation in Algeria,[36] the UAE[37] and Yemen.[33] The reason for the rising trend in consanguinity has been attributed to the increase in the availability of cousins due to high fertility.[33]

Consanguinity and reproductive health

While the concept of inheritance is not clear in the minds of many lay people, consanguinity is linked to high incidences of congenital malformations, mental retardation and disability. Studies indicate that in populations where the practice of inbred marriages is high, the frequency of homozygosity for autosomal conditions and the incidence of congenital anomalies, abortions, stillbirths and early childhood deaths are likely to rise.[3,38] The reason behind this observation is that the more closely two people are related, the more genes they share. A marriage between first cousins increases the risk of having a child with a severe congenital or genetic disorder by 2.5 times since parents share one-eighth of their genes. An average of 30% first cousin marriages in a population would increase the birth prevalence of many conditions by 5–15 times and their collective frequency by 5.5 times. Frequent consanguineous marriage increases the incidence of autosomal recessive disorders by 5–10 times at the population level. When first cousin marriage is considered, the risk of recessively inherited disorders is multiplied by 15–30 times; hence, there is a doubling of the total frequency of congenital and genetic disorders.[39]

While the incidence of recessively inherited disorders increases with the increasing trend of consanguineous marriages, consanguinity has no effect on the frequency of autosomal dominant or X-linked conditions. Autosomal dominant conditions result from just one copy of a deleterious mutation. Thus, having two parents with the same autosomal dominant mutation does not make an individual more susceptible than someone with only one affected parent. Similarly, just one copy of a deleterious X-linked recessive mutation will result in disease in males. Hence, having related parents does not increase the risk of a male with X-linked recessive disease.

Recently, many studies from the region have drawn strong correlations between consanguinity and hearing loss,[40] death rates in children,[41] respiratory allergies, eczema,[42] congenital heart defects,[43] mental retardation, epilepsy, diabetes[44] and many other conditions.[1,2]

Arab family structure and transmission genetics

The extended family structure, commonly present in Arab societies and mostly associated with consanguinity, tends to display unique distribution patterns for genetic diseases that are not present in many other societies. A major model that explains this concept is the vertical dissemination of a genetic mutation in an Arab or in a Western family. In the typical Western family, carriers of mutations usually become scattered through the general population through marriage. After a few generations, their genetic relationship to each other is unrecognized, therefore a family history suggesting a genetic basis for their predisposition to certain disease states is easily missed. On the other hand, in an Arab society mutation carriers mostly remain concentrated within the extended family, and the genetic nature of their disease predisposition is often much more obvious.

The economic impact of genetic disorders

Genetic disorders are chronic in nature and often require lifelong management with no definitive cure. In the Arab world, several disorders, including chromosomal (Down syndrome, Turner syndrome), single-gene (sickle cell disease, thalassemia, glucose-6-phosphate dehydrogenase deficiency, hemophilia, inborn errors of metabolism) and multifactorial disorders (coronary artery disease, arteriosclerosis, diabetes mellitus, hypertension, obesity) are common. Some of these disorders have assumed epidemic proportions, as in the cases of sickle cell disease, alpha-thalassemia, hypertension and diabetes mellitus. The impact of each of these disorders differs according to their severity, but many of them have medical, surgical or cosmetic consequences. Often, these conditions result in spontaneous abortion, neonatal death, and increased morbidity and mortality in both children and adults. They are a significant healthcare and psychosocial burden for the patient, the family, the healthcare system and the community as a whole.[45]

In terms of economic burden, patients with genetic or partly genetic disorders have longer and more frequent hospital admissions with a higher number of surgeries than do other patients.[46,47] Additionally, the total costs paid by patients with genetic conditions are slightly greater,[48] and these patients often must travel significant distances to get specialized treatment.[46]

In recent years, heath economists have made significant advances in calculating the costs of genetic disorders, as well as disabilities caused by various congenital abnormalities. There are now generally accepted "cost of illness" estimates for all common genetic conditions:

➡ *beta-thalassemia:* treatment of beta-thalassemia major is currently an expensive option and has great financial implications for any health authority where the disease is highly prevalent. The total lifetime (up to 60 years of age) treatment costs of a patient with beta-thalassemia are estimated to be $416 000; thus, an average of about $7000 annually.[49]

•◦ *sickle cell disease:* Davis and colleagues[50] estimated the direct cost of each hospitalization associated with sickle cell disease to be $6300. Patients with sickle cell disease are frequent users of healthcare services. On average, a sickle cell disease patient is subject to one hospital admission per year and eight outpatient visits annually.[51] Although much of the treatment cost is covered by governments or supported by non-governmental organizations in the region, this may be changing in some regions. Additionally, many of the patients must travel long distances, and this adds to the overall cost of treatment.

•◦ *cystic fibrosis:* studies have shown that hospitalization costs for patients with cystic fibrosis vary according to the severity of their disease. However, economists have estimated that the total cost per person with cystic fibrosis to be about $285 000 over their lifetime,[52] with an annual average of about $9400 per patient, of which 28% of total cost is attributable to drug costs.[53]

•◦ *hemophilia:* like other genetic disorders, hemophilia is a lifelong condition which results in profound physical, emotional, economic and social problems for those afflicted. The severity of bleeding episodes is correlated with the degree of deficiency of the Factor VIII protein in the blood. Accordingly, hemophiliacs suffer from mild, moderate or severe disease. Medical expenses vary among patients according to the severity of the deficiency. In the moderate-to-severe group, one study from 1972 estimated medical expenses to exceed $1000 per year.[54] Hemophiliacs may be denied health insurance, thus shifting the costs to the family.

•◦ *congenital bilateral permanent childhood hearing impairment:* a recent study estimating the economic costs of bilateral permanent childhood hearing impairment (PCHI) in the preceding year of life for children seven to nine years of age found that the mean societal cost was about $26 700 per child, compared to $8000 in children with normal hearing.[55]

In 1995, Waitzman and colleagues estimated that the total economic cost of cerebral palsy, spina bifida, truncus arteriosus, single ventricle, transposition/double outlet right ventricle, tetralogy of fallot, tracheo-esophageal fistula, colorectal atresia, cleft lip or palate, atresia/stenosis of the small intestine, renal agenesis, urinary obstruction, lower limb reduction, upper limb reduction, omphalocele, gastroschisis, Down syndrome, and diaphragmatic hernia in the United States was $10.8 billion (2004 normalized data) for a single year's cohort. This total cost comprises $2.8 billion in direct healthcare costs and $8 billion in indirect costs such as developmental services, special education and lost productivity. If we extrapolate these numbers adjusting for the differences in population between the United States and all Arab countries, and ignore the fact that many of these 18 birth defects occur more frequently in Arab countries than elsewhere, then the cost of these problems in Arab countries is about $13 billion per year.

Preventive aspects of genetic disorders

The successful management of genetic disorders also incurs a high financial cost, which could be eased by the application of effective prevention programs in populations at risk of genetic disease.[56] Prevention programs are effective in decreasing the impact of genetic disorders on families and societies and also lead to early treatment and improvements in outcome and prognosis.[57] A majority of Arab countries have the expertise and resources to apply most of these preventive measures, especially in the areas of newborn screening and carrier screening for prevalent genetic disorders. However, having the technology and resources alone is not enough to start effective programs. For example, population screening should be performed only if the abnormal finding in question can change the clinical management, and if this management will improve the prognosis. Economic considerations are also a factor; the cost of screening should justify the financial savings and emotional impact involved in detecting affected individuals. In addition, no genetic screening program will be successful if it is not accompanied by extensive educational activities aimed at both the general public and healthcare providers to aid effective participation.[58] Furthermore, these programs are most successful when they are sensitive to the cultural backgrounds of populations in which they are applied.[59]

Genetic disorders in Arab populations

The *Catalogue for Transmission Genetics in Arabs* (CTGA) database is a continuously updated catalogue of bibliographic material and observations on human gene variants and inherited, or heritable, genetic diseases in Arab individuals. The database is maintained by the Centre for Arab Genomic Studies (www.cags.org.ae). Since the public release of the CTGA database in 2004, our knowledge about genetic disorders in Arab populations continues to expand. This process is largely driven by various methods used at the Centre for Arab Genomic Studies (CAGS) to collect data and information on genetic conditions in Arab patients.[1]

As of May 2007, the CTGA database has recorded the presence of 816 phenotype/disease entries in Arab individuals. However, data on only about 300 related genes are available in the CTGA database. This is a reflection of the fact that clinical observation is emphasized over molecular analysis in most of the research conducted in the region. The majority of disease records in the database come from the UAE [241], Saudi Arabia [148], Palestine [127], Lebanon [125], Bahrain [120], Tunisia [94], Egypt [92], Kuwait [83], Morocco [77], and Oman [67]. This distribution is highly preliminary since CAGS has carried out extensive surveys to define the extent of genetic disorders in the UAE (2004–05) and Bahrain (2006–07). Very recently, a new survey was launched in Oman and is due for completion in early 2008. On the other hand, data from other Arab countries have been collected through limited reviews of international bibliographic indices as well as paper submissions from their corresponding authors. It is anticipated that in the coming five to ten years major surveys will be conducted in other Arab countries to obtain a more accurate picture of the extent of genetic disorders in the Arab world.

Classification and molecular complexity of genetic disorders in Arab populations

By employing the World Health Organization *International Classification of Disease,* version 10 (ICD-10), it is possible to categorize the distribution of genetic disorders in the Arab world according to disease taxonomies. Just over one-third of genetic disorders in Arab individuals result from congenital malformations and chromosomal abnormalities (34.6%). These are then followed by endocrine and metabolic disorders (17.8%) and diseases of the nervous system (9.9%). Other types of disorders seem to occur at lower frequencies in Arab populations (*see* Figure 4.2); these findings may be due to a relative lack of specific regional research or expertise in these areas.

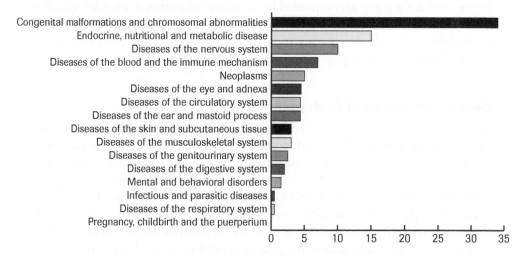

FIGURE 4.2 Classification of genetic disorders in Arabs according to the ICD-10

A detailed analysis of the molecular basis of defined genetic diseases indicates that just over half of the genetic disorders described in Arabs (54%) result from single-gene or gene loci alterations. Hence, in the presence of the necessary technical infrastructure, diagnostic services for people at risk and preventive programs may be applicable in many Arab communities.

The overwhelming proportion of genetically transmitted diseases in Arab patients are inherited through autosomal recessive modes (approximately 64%). These are followed by autosomal dominant (26%) and X-linked traits (6%). High consanguinity rates and extended family structure, which are common in Arab societies, are likely explanations for these phenomena.[1] Observations in support of this view include data from the UAE indicating that autosomal recessive and dominant disorders comprise 56% and 33%, respectively, of all genetic disorders, with 50.5% of marriages being consanguineous.[37] On the other hand, the rate of autosomal recessive disorders decreases to 37% – compared to 45% for autosomally dominant disorders – in Bahrain, where the rate of consanguineous marriage is considerably lower, at 39%.[7]

The spectrum of genetic disorders in Arab populations

A recent introduction to the CTGA database is the ability to classify genetic disorders according to their incidence rates in the Arab world. Noteworthy are two groups of disorders:

- genetic disorders that are highly prevalent and occur at annual incidences (> 100 cases per 100 000 live births). This group encompasses all hemoglobin disorders (thalassemias, sickle cell disease and hemoglobin variants), glucose-6-phosphate dehydrogenase deficiency, Down syndrome, breast cancer, diabetes, anencephaly, Graves disease, Caffey disease, Takayasu arteritis, polycystic kidneys, and other ailments.
- many other disorders do occur in the Arab world at higher incidence rates when compared to data from the rest of the world. For example: tetralogy of fallot, familial Mediterranean fever, deafness, Noonan syndrome and ankylosing spondylitis.

Many of these disorders have been extensively researched and reported in the literature, reflecting their widespread presence in Arab populations. The overwhelming distribution of these diseases in Arabs is best explained by the exposure of Arab countries to common environmental factors that encouraged natural selection for these disorders such as malaria in the case of hemoglobinopathies, and dietary traditions in the case of glucose-6-phosphate dehydrogenase deficiency.

Other genetic disorders exhibit wide geographic distributions encompassing one or more neighboring regions, such as in the cases of the hemolytic-uremic syndrome and ankylosing spondylitis. Many genetic disorders indexed in the CTGA database exhibit sporadic distribution patterns over geographically distinct regions in the Arab world. These observations strongly advocate for more regional research on these disorders to complete the picture. Candidate disorders for further research might include: alpha-thalassemia, cystic fibrosis, familial Mediterranean fever, autosomal recessive polycystic kidney disease, anencephaly, Hirschsprung disease, and others.

On the other hand, some genetic diseases exhibit specific geographic distributions. Examples include:

- *the Maghreb region:* type II bare lymphocyte syndrome and the alpha erythrocytic 1 spectrin defect
- *North Africa:* type 2C of limb-girdle muscular dystrophy
- *the Middle East:* dyssegmental dwarfism

●○ *the Arabian Gulf:* Laurence-Moon syndrome, suppressor of tumorigenicity type 8 defect, and type I primary hyperoxaluria.

It is important to note that many new syndromes and variants have recently been described in Arab people. In many cases, Arab scholars and researchers were the first to describe some of these disorders, for example: the Teebi type of hypertelorism,[60] the Teebi-Shaltout syndrome,[61] Al-Gazali syndrome[62] and Megarbane syndrome.[63] Also, some genetic disorders seem to be specific to Arab populations, such as: the Lebanese type of mannose 6-phosphate receptor recognition defect,[64] the Algerian type of spondylometaphyseal dysplasia,[65] the Kuwaiti type of cardioskeletal syndrome,[66] the Yemenite deaf-blind hypopigmentation syndrome,[67] the Nablus mask-like facial syndrome,[68] the Jerash type of the distal hereditary motor neuropathy,[69] Karak syndrome[70] and the Omani type of spondyloepiphyseal dysplasia.[71]

Final notes

At present, congenital malformations are the second leading cause of infant mortality in countries of the Gulf Cooperation Council, including Bahrain, Kuwait, Oman and Qatar. Reports from Saudi Arabia indicate that congenital malformations account for about 30% of perinatal deaths.[72] Additionally, in most Arab populations the birth prevalence of severe recessively inherited disorders may approach that of congenital malformations.[39]

Approximately 36% of reported genetic disorders in Arabs remain confined to clinical observations with no significant attempts to depict their molecular pathologies. A large number of these disorders are confined to local families and communities and have not been described elsewhere. Mummifying these disorders at the clinical level represents a very serious loss for the global scientific community, since permanently burying information regarding hundreds or thousands of human gene variants might result in the loss of important information that could be used in future research, potentially leading to cures for genetically transmitted conditions. Unfortunately, no established system is yet available in many Arab medical research institutions to translate clinical observations into genetic data. The limited examples available in the Arab world are usually local efforts by medical practitioners and clinical geneticists who have developed a particular interest or have specialized in molecular studies. Increasing the emphasis on subjects such as molecular genetics in medical schools in the region will help to create future generations of physicians and other medical personnel capable of establishing the phenotype–genotype correlations that are key elements in modern medical applications of genetics.

Databasing prevalence data, in addition to the molecular pathologies leading to genetic disorders in Arabs, offers a solid groundwork to promote enhanced education in the field and employ knowledge-driven development to address urgent regional health needs. The organization of such information also promotes Arab scientists to a position of strength and allows them to contribute to global research efforts in the field and build sustainable research activities based upon education and the improvement of human health.[73]

References

1 Tadmouri G. Genetic disorders in Arab populations: a 2006 update. In: Tadmouri G, Al Ali M, Al Khaja N, editors. *Genetic Disorders in the Arab World: Bahrain.* Dubai; 2006.

2 Tadmouri G. The Arab world. In: Tadmouri G, Al Ali M, Al Khaja N, editors. *Genetic Disorders in the Arab World: United Arab Emirates.* Dubai; 2004.

3 El-Hazmy M, Warsy A. Genetic disorders among Arab populations. *Saudi Medical Journal* 1996; **17:** 108–23.

4 Anon. *World Almanac Book of Facts.* USA; 2006.

5 Benallegue A, Kedji F. Consanguinité et santé publique: une étude algérienne. *Arch Fr Pédiatr* 1984; **41 (6):** 435–40.

6 Enquête nationale algérienne sur la fécondité en familles, femmes et contraception. In: Kouaouci A, editor. *Contribution des Nations Unies pour la Population et Centre National d'Etudes et d'Analyses pour la Planification;* 1992.

7 Al-Arrayed SS. Review of the spectrum of genetic diseases in Bahrain. *East Mediterr Health J* 1999; **5 (6):** 1114–20.

8 Hafez M, El-Tahan H, Awadalla M *et al.* Consanguineous matings in the Egyptian population. *J Med Genet* 1983; **20 (1):** 58–60.

9 Egypt National Population Council. *Demographic and Health Survey 1988.* Cairo: National Population Council; 1989.

10 Al-Hamamy H, Al-Bayati N, Al-Kubaisy W. Consanguineous marriages in Iraqi urban population and the effect on pregnancy outcome and infant mortality. *Iraqi Medical Journal* 1986; **34:** 76–80.

11 Khoury SA, Massad D. Consanguineous marriage in Jordan. *Am J Med Genet* 1992; **43 (5):** 769–75.

12 Al-Nasser K, Kelly C, El-Kazimi A. Patterns of consanguinity in the population of Kuwait. *Am J Hum Genet* 1989; **45 (Suppl 4).**

13 Al-Awadi SA, Moussa MA, Naguib KK *et al.* Consanguinity among the Kuwaiti population. *Clin Genet* 1985; **27 (5):** 483–6.

14 Klat M, Khudr A. Religious endogamy and consanguinity in marriage patterns in Beirut, Lebanon. *Soc Biol* 1986; **33 (1–2):** 138–45.

15 Broadhead R, Sehgal K. Consanguinity and congenital anomalies in East Libya. *Garyounis Medical Journal* 1981; **4 (1):** 3–6.

16 National Statistical Office. *Mauritania Maternal and Child Health Survey (1990–91).* Islamic Republic of Mauritania and the League of Arab States; 1992.

17 Hammami A, Elgazzeh M, Chalbi N *et al.* Endogamy and consanguinity in Mauritania. *Tunis Med* 2005; **83 (1):** 38–42.

18 Azelmat M, Ayad M, Belhachmi H. *Enquête nationale sur la planification familiale et de la santé de la population au Maroc.* Rabat: Ministère de la santé publique, Services des études et de l'information sanitaire; 1987.

19 Azelmat M, Ayad M, Housni E. *Enquête nationale sur la population et la santé (ENPS-II).* Rabat: Ministère de la santé publique; 1992.

20 Sulaiman AJ, Al-Riyami A, Farid S *et al.* Oman Family Health Survey 1995. *J Trop Pediatr* 2001; **47 Suppl 1:** 1–33.

21 Rajab A, Patton MA. A study of consanguinity in the Sultanate of Oman. *Ann Hum Biol* 2000; **27 (3):** 321–6.

22 Jaber L, Merlob P, Bu X *et al.* Marked parental consanguinity as a cause for increased major malformations in an Israeli Arab community. *Am J Med Genet* 1992; **44 (1):** 1–6.

23 Ministry of Health. *Qatar Family Health Survey.* State of Qatar; 1999.

24 Bener A, Alali KA. Consanguineous marriage in a newly developed country: the Qatari population. *J Biosoc Sci* 2006; **38 (2):** 239–46.

25 Wong SS, Anokute CC. The effect of consanguinity on pregnancy outcome in Saudi Arabia. *J R Soc Health* 1990; **110 (4):** 146–7.

26 El-Hazmi MA, al-Swailem AR, Warsy AS *et al.* Consanguinity among the Saudi Arabian population. *J Med Genet* 1995; **32 (8):** 623–6.

27 Saha N, Hamad RE, Mohamed S. Inbreeding effects on reproductive outcome in a Sudanese population. *Hum Hered* 1990; **40 (4):** 208–12.

28 Prothro ET, Diab LN. *Changing Family Patterns in the Arab East.* [Beirut]: American University of Beirut; 1974.

29 Aloui T, Ayad M, Habib F. *Enquête démographique et de santé en Tunisie.* Tunisie: Office national de la famille et de la population; 1988.

30 Kerkeni E, Monastiri K, Saket B *et al.* Association among education level, occupation status, and consanguinity in Tunisia and Croatia. *Croat Med J* 2006; **47 (4):** 656–61.

31 Fahmy N, Benson P, Al-Garrah D. Consanguinity in UAE: prevalence and analysis of some risk factors. *Emirates Medical Journal* 1993; **1:** 39–41.

32 Al-Gazali LI, Dawodu AH, Sabarinathan K *et al.* The profile of major congenital abnormalities in the United Arab Emirates (UAE) population. *J Med Genet* 1995; **32 (1):** 7–13.

33 Jurdi R, Saxena PC. The prevalence and correlates of consanguineous marriages in Yemen: similarities and contrasts with other Arab countries. *J Biosoc Sci* 2003; **35 (1):** 1–13.

34 Gunaid AA, Hummad NA, Tamim KA. Consanguineous marriage in the capital city Sana'a, Yemen. *J Biosoc Sci* 2004; **36 (1):** 111–21.

35 Khlat M, Halabi S, Khudr A *et al.* Perception of consanguineous marriages and their genetic effects among a sample of couples from Beirut. *Am J Med Genet* 1986; **25 (2):** 299–306.

36 Zaoui S, Biemont C. Frequency of consanguineous unions in the Tlemcen area (West Algeria). *Sante* 2002; **12 (3):** 289–95.

37 Al-Gazali LI, Bener A, Abdulrazzaq YM *et al.* Consanguineous marriages in the United Arab Emirates. *J Biosoc Sci* 1997; **29 (4):** 491–7.

38 Hoodfar E, Teebi AS. Genetic referrals of Middle Eastern origin in a western city: inbreeding and disease profile. *J Med Genet* 1996; **33 (3):** 212–15.

39 Alwan A, Modell B. *Hereditary Disorders in the Eastern Mediterranean Region: role of customary consanguineous marriage.* EMRO Technical Publications Series 24. Alexandria, Egypt: WHO; 1997.

40 Bener A, Eihakeem AA, Abdulhadi K. Is there any association between consanguinity and hearing loss? *Int J Pediatr Otorhinolaryngol* 2005; **69 (3):** 327–33.

41 Hammami A, Chalbi N, Ben Abdallah M *et al.* Effects of consanguinity and social factors on mortality and fertility in Mauritania. *Tunis Med* 2005; **83 (4):** 221–6.

42 Bener A, Janahi I. Association between childhood atopic disease and parental atopic disease in a population with high consanguinity. *Coll Anthropol* 2005; **29 (2):** 677–82.

43 Yunis K, Mumtaz G, Bitar F *et al.* Consanguineous marriage and congenital heart defects: a case-control study in the neonatal period. *Am J Med Genet A* 2006; **140 (14):** 1524–30.

44 Bener A, Hussain R. Consanguineous unions and child health in the State of Qatar. *Paediatr Perinat Epidemiol* 2006; **20 (5):** 372–8.

45 Al-Hazmi M. Spectrum of genetic disorders and the impact on health care delivery: an introduction. *East Mediterr Health J* 1999; **5 (6):** 1104–13.

46 Carnevale A, Hernandez M, Reyes R *et al.* The frequency and economic burden of genetic disease in a pediatric hospital in Mexico City. *Am J Med Genet* 1985; **20 (4):** 665–75.

47 McCandless SE, Brunger JW, Cassidy SB. The burden of genetic disease on inpatient care in a children's hospital. *Am J Hum Genet* 2004; **74 (1):** 121–7.

48 Hall JG, Powers EK, McIlvaine RT *et al.* The frequency and financial burden of genetic disease in a pediatric hospital. *Am J Med Genet* 1978; **1 (4):** 417–36.

49 Karnon J, Zeuner D, Brown J *et al.* Lifetime treatment costs of beta-thalassaemia major. *Clin Lab Haematol* 1999; **21 (6):** 377–85.

50 Davis H, Moore RM, Jr, Gergen PJ. Cost of hospitalizations associated with sickle cell disease in the United States. *Public Health Rep* 1997; **112 (1):** 40–3.

51 Nietert PJ, Abboud MR, Zoller JS *et al.* Costs, charges, and reimbursements for persons with sickle cell disease. *J Pediatr Hematol Oncol* 1999; **21 (5):** 389–96.

52 Nielsen R, Gyrd-Hansen D. Prenatal screening for cystic fibrosis: an economic analysis. *Health Econ* 2002; **11 (4):** 285–99.

53 Schreyogg J, Hollmeyer H, Bluemel M *et al.* Hospitalisation costs of cystic fibrosis. *Pharmacoeconomics* 2006; **24 (10):** 999–1009.

54 Meyers RD, Adams W, Dardick K *et al.* The social and economic impact of hemophilia – a survey of 70 cases in Vermont and New Hampshire. *Am J Public Health* 1972; **62 (4):** 530–5.

55 Schroeder L, Petrou S, Kennedy C *et al.* The economic costs of congenital bilateral permanent childhood hearing impairment. *Pediatrics* 2006; **117 (4):** 1101–12.

56 World Health Organization. *Control of Hereditary Diseases.* Report of a WHO Scientific Group. World Health Organization; 1996.

57 Al-Odaib AN, Abu-Amero KK, Ozand PT *et al.* A new era for preventive genetic programs in the Arabian Peninsula. *Saudi Med J* 2003; **24 (11):** 1168–75.

58 Khalifa MM. Preventive aspects of genetic morbidity: experiences of the Canadian model. *East Mediterr Health J* 1999; **5 (6):** 1121–8.

59 Meyer BF. Strategies for the prevention of hereditary diseases in a highly consanguineous population. *Ann Hum Biol* 2005; **32 (2):** 174–9.

60 Teebi AS. New autosomal dominant syndrome resembling craniofrontonasal dysplasia. *Am J Med Genet* 1987; **28 (3):** 581–91.

61 Teebi AS, Shaltout AA. Craniofacial anomalies, abnormal hair, camptodactyly, and caudal appendage. *Am J Med Genet* 1989; **33 (1):** 58–60.

62 Al Gazali LI, al Talabani J, Mosawi A, Lytle W. Anterior segment anomalies of the eye, clefting and skeletal abnormalities in two sibs of consanguineous parents: Michels syndrome or new syndrome? *Clin Dysmorphol* 1994; **3 (3):** 238–44.

63 Megarbane A, Ruchoux MM, Loeys B *et al.* Short stature, abnormal face, joint laxity, dislocation, hernias, delayed bone age, and severe psychomotor retardation in two

brothers: previously undescribed MCA/MR syndrome. *Am J Med Genet* 2001; **104 (3):** 221–4.

64 Alexander D, Dudin G, Talj F *et al.* Five related Lebanese individuals with high plasma lysosomal hydrolases: a new defect in mannose-6-phosphate receptor recognition? *Am J Hum Genet* 1984; **36 (5):** 1001–14.

65 Kozlowski K, Bacha L, Massen R *et al.* A new type of spondylo-metaphyseal dysplasia – Algerian type: report of five cases. *Pediatr Radiol* 1988; **18 (3):** 221–6.

66 Reardon W, Hurst J, Farag TI *et al.* Two brothers with heart defects and limb shortening: case reports and review. *J Med Genet* 1990; **27 (12):** 746–51.

67 Warburg M, Tommerup N, Vestermark S *et al.* The Yemenite deaf-blind hypopigmentation syndrome: a new oculo-dermato-auditory syndrome. *Ophthalmic Paediatr Genet* 1990; **11 (3):** 201–7.

68 Teebi AS. Nablus mask-like facial syndrome. *Am J Med Genet* 2000; **95 (4):** 407–8.

69 Christodoulou K, Zamba E, Tsingis M *et al.* A novel form of distal hereditary motor neuronopathy maps to chromosome 9p21.1-p12. *Ann Neurol* 2000; **48 (6):** 877–84.

70 Mubaidin A, Roberts E, Hampshire D *et al.* Karak syndrome: a novel degenerative disorder of the basal ganglia and cerebellum. *J Med Genet* 2003; **40 (7):** 543–6.

71 Rajab A, Kunze J, Mundlos S. Spondyloepiphyseal dysplasia Omani type: a new recessive type of SED with progressive spinal involvement. *Am J Med Genet A* 2004; **126 (4):** 413–19.

72 Hamamy H, Alwan A. Hereditary disorders in the Eastern Mediterranean region. *Bull World Health Organ* 1994; **72 (1):** 145–54.

73 Axton M. The germinating seed of Arab genomics. *Natural Genetics* 2006; **38 (8):** 851.

PART 2

The family

The family

CHAPTER 5

The Arab family: formation, function and dysfunction

(★ Arwa K Abdul-Haq

Introduction

The family is the basic social group which is united through bonds of kinship and marriage, and provides its members with protection, companionship, security and socialization. The structure of the family varies in different societies. The nuclear family that consists of two parents and their children is the primary unit in some societies. In other societies, the nuclear family is subordinate to the extended family, which includes the grandparents and other relatives.

Family is central to Arab society. Despite modern developments – such as increased mobility, urbanization and industrialization – that appear to be straining the traditional family, the family remains the primary support system, especially in the Arab world.[1] Emotional bonds as well as traditional collective values and loyalty to kin appear to be important in maintaining the connection with the extended family, even in the absence of common residence or geographic proximity. Several studies from Lebanon, which is considered to be one of the more Westernized Arab countries, found that the family is perceived there to be the most important of all social institutions.[2]

A study that surveyed a sample of Grade 12 students living in Arab villages, Arab towns and mixed (Muslim, Christian and Jewish) towns explored Arab adolescents' rankings of levels of commitment to their own self-development, their families, their extended family, the Arab people, and their village. It found that the most common pattern of commitment, shared by about a quarter of the respondents, was: the Arab people, followed by the respondent's family, their village, their hamula (clan) and, finally, their own self-development. Adolescents who lived in mixed towns were more likely to place self-development before that of their families or people. The second most common pattern observed placed self-development first, followed by family, village, people and hamula. There was no gender difference in the response patterns. The authors concluded that the responses represented the effects of transition from collectivist to individualistic values that Arab adolescents acquire through contact with Western-style cultures.[3]

Islam is the major religious tradition in Arab societies. It expanded the tribal pre-Islamic notion of the family to that of the *umma*, considering all Muslims and members of society brothers and sisters.[4] Yet it emphasized the family as an independent unit and made it a religious duty for each member to contribute to the support and maintenance of the family; and required the children to honor and obey their parents. Other religious traditions in the area are not dissimilar in outlook. Studies from Lebanon, Egypt and Jordan have found that Christian and Muslim families are more alike than different in their functioning and value systems.[5–8]

This chapter will start with a discussion of the concept of family structure, especially as it pertains to Arab society. This will be followed by a discussion of theories of family function and a review of the relevant literature on the Arab family. The last section will cover parenting, childrearing and socialization functions of the family.

Family structure and function

The Arab family is often described as being extended, hierarchical and male dominated.[9] The term "extended family" traditionally refers to living arrangements where more than one generation of the family live in the same household. Many researchers have found that this family structure is becoming less common as urbanization and industrialization cause the nuclear family to move away from the family of origin.[10] The notion of the predominance of extended family in the Arab world has thus been challenged. Research has documented that the traditionally defined extended family comprises a minority in both rural and urban Egypt, Syria, Sudan, Libya, Jordan, Bahrain and Kuwait.[11] However, in most Arab countries, emotional and sometimes economic bonds continue to strongly influence decision-making even in the absence of a common residence or physical proximity. In this sense, the Arab family continues to be predominantly extended.[2,12,13] In addition, some investigators have concluded that this strong relationship between the immediate family and the kin network has not been affected in any substantial way by modernization or urbanization.[11]

The term "hierarchy" refers to the chain of command in the family. It indicates different levels of authority for family members, with the father having the highest authority in the household in the Arab family. Hierarchy also indicates boundaries between individuals in different levels of authority, regulating their communication and interaction. A form of hierarchy is present in all families.[14] The hierarchical structure in Arab families appears to be different from those in societies where the conjugal family is the norm. In the Arab family, as a rule, the mother is closer to the children and does not have the same decision-making authority in family matters as does the father. Often the mother mediates between the children and the father and advocates for them.[15] This contrasts with the "typical" conjugal family where both parents have equivalent authority and constitute a subsystem separate from the children.

This dynamic may have implications for children's health. One study found that, in a sample of Jordanian women, maternal autonomy and position within the household power structure correlated positively with the children's nutritional status.[16]

The disruption of the hierarchical structure of the family may result in family dysfunction and emotional and behavioral problems in the children, in characteristic and well-described ways.[14] One common dysfunction seen in families is termed "triangulation" and refers to the situation where a third person, frequently a child, is drawn into a conflict between two people, usually the parents. For example, a couple with a distant or unfulfilling relationship can focus their attention on a symptomatic child to avoid fighting with each other. Another example is when the mother becomes over-involved with one or more of her children to compensate for an emotionally or physically absent husband. This over-involvement further alienates the husband and disrupts the hierarchy of the family, thereby decreasing parental authority. Some studies found that boundary disturbances in the family predict symptoms of depression, anxiety and attention deficit and hyperactivity disorder (ADHD) in middle childhood.[17]

Family conflict

Literature from Western countries provides ample evidence of the association of family conflict with child behavioral and emotional problems, independent of other factors.[18,19] Literature from Arab countries is scarce in this area except for some studies that document the negative effect of polygamous marriages on children, probably mediated through family conflict.[20-22]

Intergenerational conflict has been addressed in the Arab literature and has been associated or blamed for precipitating many forms of psychological suffering, mental illness and substance abuse, especially alcohol abuse.[23] In Kuwait, interparental discordance in attitudes toward cultural change was found to generate conflict, particularly in the more conservative local communities and in families with a higher age gap between spouses.[24] Attitudes toward the changing roles of women are thought to underlie or generate much of the intergenerational conflict detected in these studies.

Gender differences in perceptions of family function were found by some researchers in the Arab world. A study from the United Arab Emirates (UAE) found that male adolescents perceived family function more positively did than females. The author attributed this to the dissatisfaction of girls living in a male-oriented society where male children received preferential treatment.[25]

Studies from the region of children's perceptions of family functioning have, for the most part, utilized instruments and scales that have been developed in other parts of the world. This raises the question as to their appropriateness or effectiveness in capturing data relevant to Arab society in some cases.

Parenting

The family is the psychosocial environment in which children grow. Therefore it is a critical element in their development. Abundant research has established that the family environment which includes factors such as parenting style, parental mental health, marital conflict and family stress has a significant impact on the current and future mental and emotional health and functioning of children. A recent literature review from the United States concluded that the evidence supports the presence of a significant, enduring and protective effect of positive parenting on adolescent development. In particular, it was found that parental monitoring, open parent–child communication, supervision and a high quality of parent–child relationship deter high-risk behavior.[26]

Parenting style

Parenting style in Arab families is often described as authoritarian. This description is based on a classification of parenting styles from two observational studies conducted in the United States.[27,28] According to this research, parenting styles were classified into three types: authoritarian, authoritative and permissive. Studies in Western literature have shown that authoritarian parenting attitudes were associated with child maladjustment and behavior problems.[29] However, studies carried out in collective cultures do not show this to be the case.[30] This is thought to be due to the fact that, in collective cultures, authoritarian parenting is the norm and it is not associated with negative cognitive or emotional attitudes toward the child. Authoritarian styles of childrearing serve to teach the habit of giving priority to the welfare of the group over personal interest; this is a core value in collective societies. This observation provides evidence that parental emotions and attitudes toward the child, regardless of parenting style, are most critical to the development of self-esteem.

A study looking at parenting style and its effects on individuation and mental health of Egyptian adolescents found differences that depended on the gender of the child, and between rural and urban families. Parenting was found to be more authoritarian toward males in rural areas and toward females in urban areas. In this study, the authors found that female adolescents had higher emotional, functional and financial connectedness with their families in both rural and urban areas. The authors also found higher levels of identity problems, anxiety and depression in girls than boys, while boys showed higher levels of conduct disorders than girls. An authoritative parenting style correlated positively with connectedness and negatively with identity and conduct disorders (it was protective).[31] Another study found that while authoritative parental style correlated positively with the mental health of both gifted and non-gifted adolescents, an authoritarian style impacted negatively on the mental health of gifted but not non-gifted adolescents.[32]

Gender differences in perception of family function and parenting reflect preferential treatment of male children in the Arab family. Very little literature is available on this practice despite its prevalence and potential impact on both male and female children. A report from Yemen described the socialization process of males that promotes gender inequality and male domination. This "masculinity framework" socializes males to be strong, dominating breadwinners and guardians for their female counterparts.[33]

Some specific parenting practices have been associated with increased incidence of negative mental outcomes in the offspring, such as anxiety, depression, oppositional defiant disorder (ODD) and personality disorders.[34] However, it does seem that culture influences the effect of parenting behaviors to a large extent. For example, a study by Leung *et al.* published in *Anxiety* in 1994 found that parenting styles emphasizing others' opinions and utilizing shaming tactics were associated with higher levels of anxiety and social phobia in American but not in Chinese or Chinese American children.[35]

A study from Saudi Arabia found a positive relationship between perceived parental cruelty, overprotection, neglect and anxiety in a sample of Grade 9 and 11 students in intermediate and secondary schools in Riyadh.[36] This relationship between maternal intrusive over-involvement and negative and critical interactions has been observed in other studies in different cultures.[37] Knowledge of the vulnerability of children to psychological problems may also be low among parents in the region. A study from the UAE found low levels of adult awareness of children's vulnerability to psychological problems.[38]

Maternal mental health

Extensive literature from other world regions documents poor maternal mental health as a risk factor for childhood emotional and behavioral problems. In addition, the effects of maternal mental health problems on children tend to be long term, and extend well into adulthood. Maternal depression is associated with internalizing and externalizing behavioral problems in children.[17,39–41] Studies also document that depressed mothers find that their depressive symptoms make it difficult for them to care for their children.[42]

Maternal education

Research from the area shows inconsistent results of the effect of maternal education on children's health. A study of women with equal access to healthcare living in Israel found no significant difference in nutritional status between the children of Arab women, more than half of whom were in the lowest category of educational status, and Jewish women, only 3% of whom were in the lowest educational status category. One exception was a higher incidence of anemia in Arab children.[43] Another study from Libya found that malnutrition, stunting and wasting were all strongly associated with the mother's educational status.[44] A study from the UAE found that children with diabetes whose mothers were better educated had better self-esteem.[45]

Behavior problems in children

Behavior problems in children have traditionally been conceptualized as being either "internalizing" or "externalizing". Internalizing symptoms include depression and anxiety, sometimes referred to as emotional problems. Externalizing symptoms are primarily conduct and behavioral problems, and include aggression, non-compliance and risk-taking behavior. In addition to the difficulties that childhood behavior problems pose for the child and family, there is evidence to suggest that childhood behavioral problems are precursors of adult maladaptive behavior and mental health problems.[46-8]

Research on the epidemiology of pediatric behavioral and emotional problems has significantly increased within the past few decades with the development of valid diagnostic scales. Most of these scales have been developed in Western countries. These scales have been widely applied to research in non-Western societies. Although many of these instruments and scales are promising, there is a need to modify them to fit the different cultural constructs of behavior and establish their validity in the local setting. A study of the application of the "Strengths and Difficulties" questionnaire in a group of Arab children from Gaza strip provides a clear illustration of this problem. The study found that Western categories of mental health problems did not seem to apply to the study population. It was concluded that indigenously meaningful constructs of mental health problems needed to be developed.[49]

Western literature estimates around 20% of children have behavior problems and about half of these can be diagnosed with a specific psychiatric disorder.[50,51] A study from the UAE estimated the prevalence of behavior disorders in children to be 13.5%, with a higher prevalence among males than females (16.3% and 10.2% respectively). In this study, behavior disorders were described as emotional in 4.8% cases, conduct related in 6.9% cases and undifferentiated in 1.8% cases. In addition to female gender, very good or excellent scholastic performance and being in the middle grades [3–6] were associated with lower prevalence of behavior problems.[52] The prevalence of behavioral disorders in a sample of three-year-old children in the UAE was estimated to be 10.5% using the Pediatric Symptom checklist; this is similar to prevalence estimates from Western countries. Risk factors for disordered behavior in this study included perinatal factors, an adverse family environment, and a positive family history of mental health problems.[53]

ADHD is the most commonly diagnosed childhood behavior disorder in the Western literature. The rate of diagnosis has increased exponentially over the past two decades. ADHD is diagnosed when a child presents developmentally inappropriate levels of inattention, impulsivity and hyperactivity. These symptoms must have been evident before seven years of age and evidence of impairment must present in more than one setting (e.g. home and school). An inattentive type can be diagnosed in the absence of hyperactive symptoms and is more common in girls. Stimulant medications have proven effective in decreasing the hyperactive symptoms and improving function in these children, however, evidence is not available regarding the long term effects of treatment.

The prevalence of ADHD in a cross-sectional sample of primary school children in Qatar was estimated to be 9.4% overall. The incidence in boys was 14.1%, which was more than three-fold that of girls, at 4.4%.[54]

Chronic illness in children

The need to adopt a bio-psychosocial approach in the assessment of the child and family is especially critical in the evaluation of the child with a chronic illness or recurrent complaints, whether physical or behavioral in nature. The course of chronic illness is highly influenced by family patterns of behavior and interaction. In addition, the emotional and physical burden of caring for a child with a chronic illness has been shown to have a significant impact on both family and child. A study of a group of Kuwaiti children and adolescents with type 1 diabetes mellitus found that they had a higher prevalence of anxiety, depression and general distress than non-diabetic controls. The presence of psychological distress or symptoms of anxiety and depression were strongly correlated with poor glycemic control.[55]

Children's chronic illness, and how it affects the family

Childhood is a stage of life associated with health, growth and potential. The diagnosis of a chronic illness in the child engenders an emotional reaction that may include guilt and grief over losing normal childhood and imagined futures.[56] Feelings of guilt may be especially important if the disease is genetic or hereditary or the result of an accident that could have been prevented. Depending on the child's developmental stage, the severity of the illness and the family's reaction to the illness, some children's emotional development may be arrested.[57]

The physical burden of caring for a child with chronic illness has been shown to have consequences for maternal mental health. A study from Lebanon reported a high prevalence of depression among mothers caring for their mentally handicapped children.[58] A study from Israel found that the higher the number of informal support sources (family and friends) a mother had to assist her in caring for her disabled child, the greater well-being that she reported. In contrast, among women who utilized formal support (welfare) services, this relationship was not noted.[59]

Family dynamics that influence children's health

There is mounting evidence linking certain family interactional patterns and children's physical, emotional and psychological health. As discussed earlier, situations such as excessive family conflict, divorce and violence tend to adversely affect the emotional and mental well-being of children. In addition, the onset and or course of many physical illnesses in childhood has been shown to be influenced by family dynamics. Several patterns of family interaction have been recognized that adversely influence the course of physical illness in children. Of these, a psychosomatic family process has been described that includes triangulating behavior, overprotection, restriction of autonomy and poor conflict resolution.[14,60] For example, an acute illness such as an asthma attack in a child will temporarily bring an end to a conflict between the husband and wife as both pay attention to the sick child. This may be reinforcing to all parties including the child, who learns (usually unconsciously) that his or her being sick will stop his or her parents from fighting. Thus a pattern is created in the family where the child's illness maintains peace, but also victimizes the child and fosters helplessness.

The influence of family stress on childhood illness has been explored in a study from Egypt. A sample of Egyptian children found that non-organic recurrent abdominal pain in children was commonly associated with family troubles such as maternal illness, over-criticism, absence of the mother or father (e.g. working abroad), frequent punishment, conflict and jealousy between siblings, divorce or death of a parent. School-related problems were found in 40%, which included fear of failure, and frequent punishment by teachers.[61]

Family structure is also an important risk factor for psychological morbidity in children. Excessive fearfulness was found in 50% of a stratified random sample of 12–17-year-old children in the UAE. The presence of fears correlated positively with female gender, parental death or divorce, living with a single parent or relatives, low income or an adverse home environment.[62] This agrees with similar literature from Western countries which suggests that certain family types (stepmother, complex step-families and single-parent families) are a proxy for exposure to psychosocial risks. The extent of family influence on children's emotional and behavioral health may be strongest in high-stress settings.[63]

These findings tend to support the proposition of the concept of the "risky family", which is characterized by conflict, aggression and cold, unsupportive and neglectful relationships that can create vulnerabilities or interact with genetically based vulnerabilities in offspring to produce disruptions in psychosocial functioning.[64]

Conclusion

The family in the Arab world is a fundamental institution that is being exposed to many pressures including culture change, political conflict and increased mobility. Family dynamics influence the well-being and emotional health of all family members. Children are particularly vulnerable because of their total dependence on the family for their survival. Understanding the role that the family plays in a patient's life provides the clinician with valuable insights in understanding and managing many common behavioral and emotional problems seen in clinical practice.

Models to explain family function and dysfunction need to take into account cultural norms. Therefore, culturally relevant paradigms and tools that will help us to understand and work with families in our region should be developed.

References

1 Fernea EW. *Women and the Family in the Middle East: new voices of change*. 1st ed. Austin: University of Texas Press; 1985.

2 Kazarian SS. Family functioning, cultural orientation, and psychological well-being among university students in Lebanon. *J Soc Psychol* 2005; **145 (2):** 141–52.

3 Ben-Ari A, Azaiza F. Commitment among Arab adolescents in Israel. *Journal of Social Psychology* 1998; **138 (5):** 655–60.

4 Abudabbeh N, Hays P. Cognitive behavioral therapy with people of Arab heritage. In: Hays P, editor. *Culturally Responsive Cognitive Behavioral Therapy: assessment, practice and supervision*. Washington, DC: American Psychological Association; 2006. pp. 141–59.

5 Ali NS, Khalil HZ, Yousef W. A comparison of American and Egyptian cancer patients' attitudes and unmet needs. *Cancer Nurs* 1993; **16 (3):** 193–203.

6 Starr P. Continuity and change in social distance: studies from the Arab East – a research report. *Social Forces* 1978; **56 (4):** 1221–7.

7 Dodd P. The effect of religious affiliation on woman's role in Middle Eastern Arab society. *Journal of Comparative Family Studies* 1974; **5 (2):** 117–29.

8 Droeber J. "Woman to woman" – the significance of religiosity for young women in Jordan. *Women's Studies International Forum* 2003; **26 (5):** 409–24.

9 Al-Krenawi A. Socio-political aspects of mental health practice with Arabs in the Israeli context. *Isr J Psychiatry Relat Sci* 2005; **42 (2):** 126–36.

10 Fellous M. [Children for where?] *Temps Mod* 1981; **38 (424):** 912–39.

11 Al-Thakeb F. Size and composition of the Arab family: census and survey data. *Int J Sociol Fam* 1981; **11 (2):** 171–8.

12 Al-Thakeb F. The Arab family and modernity. Evidence from Kuwait. *Current Anthropology* 1985; **26 (5):** 575–80.

13 Farsoun S. Family structure and society in modern Lebanon. In: Sweet LE, American Museum of Natural History, editors. *Peoples and Cultures of the Middle East: an*

anthropological reader. Garden City, NY: Published for the American Museum of Natural History [by] the Natural History Press; 1970. pp. 257–307.

14 Minuchin S, Nichols MP, Lee W-Y. *Assessing Families and Couples: from symptom to system.* Boston: Pearson/Allyn and Bacon; 2007.

15 Smadi F. The Arabian family in the light of Minuchin's systematic theory: an analytical approach. *Social Behavior and Personality* 2003; **31 (5):** 467–82.

16 Doan RM, Bisharat L. Female autonomy and child nutritional status: the extended-family residential unit in Amman, Jordan. *Soc Sci Med* 1990; **31 (7):** 783–9.

17 Jacobvitz D, Hazen N, Curran M *et al.* Observations of early triadic family interactions: boundary disturbances in the family predict symptoms of depression, anxiety, and attention-deficit/hyperactivity disorder in middle childhood. *Dev Psychopathol* 2004; **16 (3):** 577–92.

18 Lucia VC, Breslau N. Family cohesion and children's behavior problems: a longitudinal investigation. *Psychiatry Res* 2006; **141 (2):** 141–9.

19 Shaw DS, Criss MM, Schonberg MA *et al.* The development of family hierarchies and their relation to children's conduct problems. *Dev Psychopathol* 2004; **16 (3):** 483–500.

20 Eapen V, al-Gazali L, Bin-Othman S *et al.* Mental health problems among schoolchildren in United Arab Emirates: prevalence and risk factors. *J Am Acad Child Adolesc Psychiatry* 1998; **37 (8):** 880–6.

21 Al-Krenawi A, Graham JR, Slonim-Nevo V. Mental health aspects of Arab-Israeli adolescents from polygamous versus monogamous families. *J Soc Psychol* 2002; **142 (4):** 446–60.

22 Slonim-Nevo V, Al-Krenawi A. Success and failure among polygamous families: the experience of wives, husbands, and children. *Fam Process* 2006; **45 (3):** 311–30.

23 El-Islam MF. Cultural change and intergenerational relationships in Arabian families. *International Journal of Family Psychiatry* 1983; **4:** 321–8.

24 El-Islam MF. Interparental differences in attitudes to cultural changes in Kuwait. *Soc Psychiatry Psychiatr Epidemiol* 1988; **23:** 109–13.

25 Alnajjar AA. Adolescents' perceptions of family functioning in the United Arab Emirates. *Adolescence* 1996; **31 (122):** 433–42.

26 DeVore ER, Ginsburg KR. The protective effects of good parenting on adolescents. *Curr Opin Pediatr* 2005; **17 (4):** 460–5.

27 Baumrind D. Effects of authoritative parental control on child behavior. *Child Development* 1966; **37 (4):** 887–907.

28 Baumrind D. Child care practices anteceding three patterns of preschool behavior. *Genetic Psychology Monographs* 1967; **75 (1):** 43–88.

29 Thompson A, Hollis C, Richards D. Authoritarian parenting attitudes as a risk for conduct problems. *European Child and Adolescent Psychiatry* 2003; **12 (6):** 320–1.

30 Rudy D, Grusec J. Authoritarian parenting in individualist and collectivist groups: associations with maternal emotion and cognition and children's self esteem. *Journal of Family Psychology* 2006; **20 (1):** 68–78.

31 Dwairy M, Menshar KE. Parenting style, individuation, and mental health of Egyptian adolescents. *J Adolesc* 2006; **29 (1):** 103–17.

32 Dwairy M. Parenting styles and mental health of Arab gifted adolescents. *Gifted Child Quarterly* 2004; **48 (4):** 275–86.

33 Elsanousi M. Strategies and approaches to enhance the role of men and boys in gender equality. In: Expert Group Meeting on the Role of Men and Boys in Achieving Gender Equality; 2003, 21–4 October 2003; Brasilia, Brazil; 2003.

34 Johnson JG, Cohen P, Chen H *et al.* Parenting behaviors associated with risk for offspring personality disorder during adulthood. *Arch Gen Psychiatry* 2006; **63 (5):** 579–87.

35 Leung AW, Heimberg RG, Holt CS *et al.* Social anxiety and perception of early parenting among American, Chinese American, and social phobic samples. *Anxiety* 1994; **1 (2):** 80–9.

36 Addelaim F. The relationship between anxiety and some parental treatment styles. *Arab Journal of Psychiatry* 2003; **14 (2):** 116–26.

37 Xia G, Qian M. The relationship of parenting style to self reported mental health among two subcultures in China. *Journal of Adolescence* 2001; **24 (2):** 251–60.

38 Swadi H, Karim L. Children's vulnerability to psychological health problems: attitudes of a community sample of Arabs in the United Arab Emirates. *Arab Journal of Psychiatry* 1997; **8 (2):** 81–6.

39 Halligan SL, Murray L, Martins C *et al.* Maternal depression and psychiatric outcomes in adolescent offspring: a 13-year longitudinal study. *J Affect Disord* 2007; **97 (1–3):** 145–54.

40 Pesonen AK, Raikkonen K, Heinonen K *et al.* Depressive vulnerability in parents and their 5-year-old child's temperament: a family system perspective. *J Fam Psychol* 2006; **20 (4):** 648–55.

41 Civic D, Holt VL. Maternal depressive symptoms and child behavior problems in a nationally representative normal birthweight sample. *Matern Child Health J* 2000; **4 (4):** 215–21.

42 Grupp-Phelan J, Whitaker RC, Naish AB. Depression in mothers of children presenting for emergency and primary care: impact on mothers' perceptions of caring for their children. *Ambul Pediatr* 2003; **3 (3):** 142–6.

43 Habib S, Rishpon S, Rubin L. Mother's education and ethnicity: effect on health measures for children in the Haifa subdistrict. *Harefuah* 2005; **144 (6):** 402–6, 455.

44 Hameida J, Billot L, Deschamps JP. Growth of preschool children in the Libyan Arab Jamahiriya: regional and sociodemographic differences. *East Mediterr Health J* 2002; **8 (4–5):** 458–69.

45 Eapen V, Mabrouk AA, Sabri S *et al.* A controlled study of psychosocial factors in young people with diabetes in the United Arab Emirates. *Ann N Y Acad Sci* 2006; **1084:** 325–8.

46 Rosenberg SD, Lu W, Mueser KT *et al.* Correlates of adverse childhood events among adults with schizophrenia spectrum disorders. *Psychiatr Serv* 2007; **58 (2):** 245–53.

47 Schilling EA, Aseltine RH, Jr, Gore S. Adverse childhood experiences and mental health in young adults: a longitudinal survey. *BMC Public Health* 2007; **7:** 30.

48 Anda RF, Brown DW, Felitti VJ *et al.* Adverse childhood experiences and prescribed psychotropic medications in adults. *Am J Prev Med* 2007; **32 (5):** 389–94.

49 Thabet AA, Stretch D, Vostanis P. Child mental health problems in Arab children: application of the strengths and difficulties questionnaire. *Int J Soc Psychiatry* 2000; **46 (4):** 266–80.

50 Zill N, Schoenborn CA. Developmental, learning, and emotional problems. Health of our nation's children, United States, 1988. *Adv Data* 1990 **190:** 1–18.

51 Brotman MA, Schmajuk M, Rich BA *et al.* Prevalence, clinical correlates, and longitudinal course of severe mood dysregulation in children. *Biol Psychiatry* 2006; **60 (9):** 991–7.

52 Al-Kuwaiti MA, Hossain MM, Absood GH. Behaviour disorders in primary school children in Al Ain, United Arab Emirates. *Ann Trop Paediatr* 1995; **15 (1):** 97–104.

53 Eapen V, Al-Sabosy M, Saeed M *et al.* Child psychiatric disorders in a primary care Arab population. *Int J Psychiatry Med* 2004; **34 (1):** 51–60.

54 Bener A, Qahtani RA, Abdelaal I. The prevalence of ADHD among primary school children in an Arabian society. *J Atten Disord* 2006; **10 (1):** 77–82.

55 Moussa MA, Alsaeid M, Abdella N *et al.* Social and psychological characteristics of Kuwaiti children and adolescents with type 1 diabetes. *Soc Sci Med* 2005; **60 (8):** 1835–44.

56 McDaniel SH, Hepworth J, Doherty WJ. *Medical Family Therapy: a biopsychosocial approach to families with health problems.* New York, NY: Basic Books; 1992.

57 Sexton TL, Weeks GR, Robbins MS. *Handbook of Family Therapy: the science and practice of working with families and couples.* New York: Brunner-Routledge; 2003.

58 Azar M, Badr LK. The adaptation of mothers of children with intellectual disability in Lebanon. *J Transcult Nurs* 2006; **17 (4):** 375–80.

59 Duvdevany I, Abboud S. Stress, social support and well-being of Arab mothers of children with intellectual disability who are served by welfare services in northern Israel. *J Intellect Disabil Res* 2003; **47 (Pt 4–5):** 264–72.

60 Nichols MP, Schwartz RC. *Family Therapy: concepts and methods.* 3rd ed. Boston: Allyn and Bacon; 1995.

61 Abd El-Mageid FY, Abou-El Fetouh AM, Abou-Hatab MF. Recurrent abdominal pain among a sample of Egyptian children in relation to family and school related problems. *J Egypt Public Health Assoc* 2002; **77 (1–2):** 201–23.

62 Mohammed NA, Eapen V, Bener A. Prevalence and correlates of childhood fears in Al-Ain, United Arab Emirates. *East Mediterr Health J* 2001; **7 (3):** 422–7.

63 O'Connor TG, Dunn J, Jenkins JM *et al.* Family settings and children's adjustment: differential adjustment within and across families. *Br J Psychiatry* 2001; **179:** 110–15.

64 Repetti RL, Taylor SE, Seeman TE. Risky families: family social environments and the mental and physical health of offspring. *Psychol Bull* 2002; **128 (2):** 330–66.

CHAPTER 6

Child abuse and neglect

(★ *Adib Essali*

Introduction

Violence is a major global public health issue. Over one million people die every year because of intentional acts of self-directed, interpersonal or collective violence. Many more are injured or suffer other non-fatal health consequences as a result of being the victim or witness to acts of violence.[1] However, in many countries, violence prevention remains a new or emerging field in public health.

Existing approaches to violence, which are mainly reactive, may be enhanced by a public health approach which is focused on changing the behavioral, social and environmental factors that give rise to violence.[2]

Public health is committed to aiding communities to solve their own health problems, and to assuring that necessary health services are available in communities. This commitment can be extended to include reducing the severity and duration of the physical or psychological injuries and disabilities caused by violent incidents. Public health can make a significant contribution to the management of violence through its focus on prevention, scientific approaches and potential to coordinate multidisciplinary efforts. It can also play a role in assuring the availability of services for victims of violence.

Violence may be defined as "the intentional use of physical force or power, threatened or actual, against oneself, another person, or against a group or community, that either results in or has a high likelihood of resulting in injury, death, psychological harm, maldevelopment or deprivation".[1] This definition encompasses all types of violence and covers the wide range of acts of commission and omission that constitute violence and outcomes beyond deaths and injuries. Violence may be categorized into self-inflicted, interpersonal and collective (*see* Figure 6.1), and each category can be subdivided to reflect specific types of violence, settings of violence, and the nature of violent acts (physical, sexual, psychological, and deprivation or neglect).

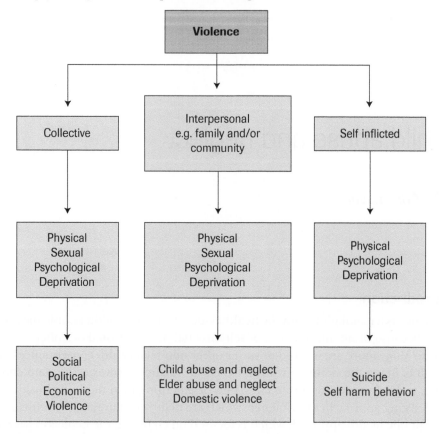

FIGURE 6.1 Category, types, settings, and nature of violence

Thus, the spectrum of violence includes child abuse and neglect by caregivers, intimate partner violence, elder abuse, self-directed violence and collective violence. While it is important for healthcare workers to be able to deal with all these types of violence, this chapter is limited to dealing with the entity of child abuse and neglect (CAN).

Definition of CAN

Every child deserves to grow up in a safe and nurturing environment.

Parents have a fundamental right to raise their children as they see fit, and society presumes that parents will act in their children's best interest. When parents do not protect their children from harm and meet their basic needs, as with cases of CAN, society has a responsibility to intervene to protect the health and welfare of these children. Any intervention in family life on behalf of children must be guided by the law and sound professional practice standards.

To prevent and respond to CAN effectively, there should be a common understanding of definitions of actions and omissions that constitute child maltreatment. Unfortunately, there is no single, universally applied definition of CAN. However, there are commonalities across definitions, and CAN may be defined as any act or failure to act on the part of a parent or caregiver that results in death, serious physical or emotional harm, sexual abuse or exploitation of a child. This definition refers specifically to parents and other caregivers, and a "child" is any person under the age of 18.

Types of CAN

There are four commonly recognized forms of child abuse or maltreatment: physical, sexual, neglect and psychological.[3]

➥ *physical abuse* is inflicting a physical injury upon a child through burning, hitting, punching, shaking, kicking, beating or otherwise harming a child. It may, sometimes, be the result of over-discipline or culturally accepted practices. While cultural practices are generally respected, healthcare workers should work with parents to discourage harmful behavior and suggest preferable alternatives.

➥ *child sexual abuse* includes a wide range of behaviors exhibited by a person responsible for the care of a child, and can involve varying degrees of violence and emotional trauma. Child sexual abuse generally refers to sexual acts, sexually motivated behaviors involving children, or sexual exploitation of children. It includes fondling, intercourse, incest, rape, sodomy, exhibitionism, sexual exploitation, or exposure to pornography. The most commonly reported cases involve incest – sexual abuse occurring among family members, including those in biological families, adoptive families and step-families. Incest most often occurs within a father–daughter relationship; however, sexual abuse may also be committed by other relatives or caretakers.

➥ *child neglect* is the failure to provide for the child's basic needs. Neglect can be physical, educational or emotional. Physical neglect can include not providing adequate food or clothing, appropriate medical care, supervision, or proper protection from the weather. Educational neglect includes failure to provide appropriate schooling, special educational needs, or allowing excessive truancies. Psychological neglect includes the lack of emotional support and love, chronic inattention to the child, or exposure to domestic violence or to drug and alcohol abuse.

➥ *psychological abuse* is a pattern of caregiver behavior that conveys to children that they are worthless, flawed, unloved, unwanted, endangered, or only of value to meeting another's needs. This can include parents or caretakers using extreme or bizarre forms of punishment or threatening or terrorizing a child. The term "psychological abuse" has also been termed emotional abuse, verbal abuse or mental abuse.

Incidence and prevalence

Although hundreds of thousands of children are subjected to CAN worldwide, reliable data on the prevalence and incidence of CAN are scarce. Incidence rates are usually drawn from data collected by child protection services, but not all countries have such services and not all CAN cases are reported. Prevalence rates are usually derived from cross-sectional or retrospective surveys.

In countries with well-developed social service agencies, the incidence of CAN seems to be fairly consistent. During the year 2000 in the USA, for example, 12 of every 1000 were victims of one or more types of CAN; 62.8% suffered neglect (an estimated annual incidence rate of 7 per 1000 children), 19.3% were physically abused, 10.1% were sexually abused, and 7.7% were victims of psychological maltreatment. About 160 000 children suffer from serious or life-threatening injures, and approximately 1400 children die from abusive injuries or neglect, in the USA every year.[4] It must be remembered here that these figures reflect the cases that have been reported to child protection agencies. An unknown number of cases may go unnoticed and/or unreported.

Less developed countries underreport CAN, probably because of the lack of social services. However, the widespread nature of CAN is clear. In 48 retrospective population surveys from around the world, the prevalence of sexual abuse during childhood was approximately 20% among women and 5–10% among men.[5] In the absence of formal statistics from Arab countries, an impression about the prevalence of CAN may be formed from the number of cases seen in forensic medicine departments and within criminal justice systems.[6,7] Available data suggest that the prevalence of CAN in Arab countries may not be much different from that in the rest of the world.[8,9,10]

CAN occurs across socioeconomic, religious, cultural, racial and ethnic groups, and there is no single known cause. Nor is there any single description that captures all families in which children are victims of CAN. Research, however, has identified four groups of risk factors or attributes commonly associated with CAN: parent or caregiver factors (attachment problems, unrealistic expectations of the child, punitive childrearing styles, parents who were themselves abused as children, psychiatric disorders among parents); family factors (family conflicts, chaotic family structure, abuse of other children in the family); child factors (children who are physically, mentally or behaviorally difficult); and environmental factors (socioeconomic stressors, social isolation and family secrecy).[11,12,13]

Consequences of CAN

Much research has shown that the health consequences of CAN are far broader than just death and injuries. Victims of CAN are at risk of psychological and behavioral problems that may last a lifetime.[14] Recent brain research has established a foundation for the neurobiological explanations for many of the physical, cognitive, social and emotional difficulties exhibited by children who experienced CAN in their early years. Ongoing CAN is typically associated with persistent stress that may drive the child's brain to strengthen the pathways among neurons involved in the fear response.[15,16] As a result, the brain may become "wired" to experience the world as hostile and uncaring, thus negatively influencing the child's later interactions, and prompting the child to become anxious, aggressive or withdrawn.[17] CAN may also inhibit the appropriate development of certain regions of the brain. A neglected infant or young child, for example, may not be exposed to stimuli that would activate important regions of the brain and strengthen cognitive pathways. If the regions responsible for emotional regulation are not activated, the child may have trouble controlling his or her emotions, behavior or social interactions.

All types of CAN may affect a child's psychological well-being.[18] While there is no single set of behaviors that is characteristic of all CAN victims, physically and sexually abused children often exhibit both internalizing and externalizing problems. In addition to obvious sequelae such as death, traumatic brain injury or disfigurement, physical abuse may result in long-term mental health consequences that include violence, criminal behavior, substance abuse, self-injurious and suicidal behavior, depression, anxiety, and other mental health problems.[19] While sexual abuse may leave no physical signs, its emotional and psychological consequences may be devastating. Reactions to sexual abuse can include post-traumatic stress disorder, depression, anxiety, anger, impaired sense of self, dissociative phenomena, suicidal behavior and inappropriate sexual behavior.[20,21] Neglect of nutritional and emotional needs of the child may result in significant developmental delays or failure to thrive.[22] Motor, fine motor, speech, language and cognitive delays have been documented. The resultant poor cognitive ability can lead to emotional and behavioral problems.

Moreover, exposure to CAN may affect an individual's health in a number of direct and indirect ways. Victims of sexual abuse, for example, may become infected with sexually transmitted diseases.[23] Women who have experienced sexual abuse are more likely to experience ongoing health problems. Adults who were maltreated as children show higher levels of many health problems not typically associated with CAN: heart disease, cancer, chronic lung disease and liver disease. The link between CAN and these diseases may be depression, which can influence the immune system and may lead to higher risk behaviors such as smoking, alcohol and drug use, and overeating.[24]

Medical assessment

The initial medical treatment of CAN victims should proceed no differently from treatment of accidentally injured children. However, additional attention should be paid to forensic data collection and to ensuring the safety of the child.

Each of the four overlapping categories of CAN (physical, psychological, sexual and deprivation) has unique characteristics and requires individual approaches to diagnosis and management. History-taking requires a compassionate yet objective approach to establish how the injury occurred. Information should be gathered from all available people separately, using open-ended, non-leading questions, particularly with younger children. Suspicion of CAN may arise from injuries' characteristics, unexplained or poorly explained injuries, injuries incompatible with the stated history, changing history, or significant delay in seeking treatment. Munchausen syndrome by proxy, or factitious disorder by proxy, is a covert, potentially lethal, form of CAN that may be difficult to detect and confirm. It describes a psychiatric illness of the mothers or caregivers who induce symptoms and fabricate illnesses in their children.[25,26]

The physically abused child typically presents with obvious injuries. It is not uncommon, however, for abused children to present with life-threatening occult head or abdominal trauma without a convincing history or visible external signs. Infants with head injuries may present with non-specific symptoms such as lethargy, irritability, persistent unexplained vomiting, apnea, coma or convulsions.[27] Abdominal trauma may be manifested by vomiting, pain, tenderness, shock and/or sepsis.

In suspected cases of child sexual abuse, the history should include questions regarding possible behavioral indicators of abuse, such as aggression, depression, suicidal behaviors, withdrawal, low self-esteem, nightmares, phobias, regression, school problems, sleep disorders, sexualized behavior, or somatic complaints such as headaches, general fatigue, abdominal pain, constipation, diarrhea, encopresis, genitourinary complaints or possible pregnancy.

If neglect is suspected, the infant's or child's history should include an evaluation of feeding and nutritional history, growth and developmental progress, environmental and psychosocial history, maternal (or caregiver) attachment, parents' (or caregivers') perceptions of the problem, and past history of CAN. The caregivers' level of concern may be discordant with the physician's level of concern. Often, a disturbance in bonding may be obvious, but signs of problems with attachment can also be subtle.

The physical examination of physically abused children may reveal a spectrum of injuries ranging from minor bruises and lacerations to severe trauma and death. Although such injuries may be the result of corporal punishment, the intent of the abuser (to inflict injury or not) is not relevant to the medical diagnosis. CAN should be suspected in cases of bruises on a non-ambulating infant, injuries in various stages of healing, multiple injuries, injuries with an obvious pattern, such as from a hand or implement, and injuries in locations usually well protected in accidents, such as the trunk, upper arms, upper legs, neck and face, and the perineal area.[28] The shape of burns or bruises may suggest a causative factor such as a hot iron or a cigarette. CAN accounts for about 30% of all childhood fractures, and for 75% of fractures during the first year of life.[29] Physical abuse may cause unexplained, severe and diffuse brain trauma in infants. The shaken baby syndrome is characterized by retinal hemorrhages, intracranial trauma and cerebral edema.

The physical examination may be normal in most cases of sexual abuse, including most cases of suspected or substantiated sexual abuse of prepubertal girls.[30] The most important determinant for sexual abuse is the child's (or a witness's) account of the incident. However, questioning the child about the incident should be avoided until appropriate interviewing can be arranged. Physical indicators that may be present are skin bruises caused by the use of force, bruises to the genital area, rectal abnormalities, hymenal abnormalities, and signs of sexually transmitted diseases.

In cases of neglect, the examination most often reveals a rather small and undernourished infant with most developmental milestones either intact or mildly delayed. Signs of severe malnutrition are seen from time to time, however. Failure to thrive should always be considered a possible presentation of child neglect.

Psychosocial evaluation

A detailed psychosocial evaluation is essential in every suspected case of CAN in order to understand the functioning of the family and the environment in which the abuse occurred. All above-mentioned CAN risk factors should be addressed through reviewing the family's current and past social history, finances and resources, living arrangements, background, attitudes and beliefs about childrearing, domestic or interpersonal violence, substance abuse, and mental health disorders including personality disorders and postpartum depression. Understanding the family structure and dynamics is also important to identifying sources of support for the child.

If CAN is suspected, the medical history should be completed by appropriate consultations. An interdisciplinary approach is vital in the assessment and care of children subjected to CAN, and in providing support for the caregiver and the child. Whenever possible, nutritionists, developmental specialists, physical or occupational therapists, social workers, psychologists, and/or psychiatrists should be involved. A careful forensic assessment is a necessity, as is reporting the case to child protection services.

Management

The most important step in the management of CAN cases is ensuring the child's safety. Inpatient care is recommended for acute traumatic injury, severe malnourishment and severe mental trauma. Hospitalization may also be necessary if the child's safety is in doubt.

In addition to establishing the diagnosis and providing the appropriate treatment, management of CAN cases also includes documentation of findings[31] and reporting to child protection agencies. Healthcare workers may also be required to make a forensic medical assessment and to give an expert court testimony. Photographic documentation of findings, clearly demonstrating the child's identity and the date of the photograph, is useful for both clinical and legal purposes. Depending on local protocols, the forensic interview may best be performed with the assistance of trained professionals because of its importance in protecting the child and prosecuting the perpetrator. The forensic interview differs from a good medical history in that it is mostly concerned with detailed answers to who, what, where and when the abuse occurred. The aim of the forensic interview is to convert a medical diagnosis (e.g. intracranial hemorrhage) into a forensic diagnosis (e.g. shaken baby syndrome).[32]

Laboratory and imaging investigations should be tailored to every child. In any child with suspicious bruising, a coagulation profile is helpful in excluding a bleeding diathesis. Hematuria may indicate kidney or urethral trauma. Occult abdominal trauma may be confirmed by liver or pancreatic function tests and a CT scan. Complete blood count may indicate internal hemorrhage, or, in other cases, detect chronic anemia in neglected and undernourished children. A full radiographic skeletal survey is indicated in any child aged two years or younger with evidence or a strong suspicion of physical abuse. In several studies, the incidence of asymptomatic fractures has been reported to be 15% in these cases.[33,34] A brain CT scan or MRI is indicated in any infant with suspicious neurological symptoms or signs, or a history of violent shaking. Dilated eye examination by an ophthalmologist is particularly important if shaken baby syndrome is suspected. Local protocols for sexually transmitted diseases, hepatitis B, and HIV prophylaxis and testing should be followed particularly in cases of sexual abuse.

In addition to the medical follow-up needs (e.g. orthopedic, surgical, neurological), victims of CAN often need child protection and mental healthcare. Without appropriate social service and mental health intervention, CAN is usually a recurrent and sometimes escalating problem.

Practitioners should report all CAN cases to local child protection agencies before a child is discharged from the hospital. Healthcare workers are among the groups of professionals required to report suspected CAN to the concerned authorities. Mandated reporting laws for CAN exist in many countries, and every physician should be familiar with local laws. In the USA, for instance, the *Child Abuse Prevention and Treatment Act* has been established to ensure that victimized children are identified and reported to appropriate authorities. While specific CAN prevention Acts may not be present in all countries, most countries, including Arab countries, do have some form of mandatory reporting legislation. The complexity of dealing with CAN cases may be simplified by establishing local institutional protocols specifying the diagnostic and therapeutic steps that are to be taken, who should be consulted, and how to notify child protection agencies.

Prevention of CAN

Healthcare workers are in a unique position to assist in the prevention of CAN because they have routine access to children and families, and because of their interest in the prevention of disease and the promotion of health and well-being. Activities that contribute to the prevention of CAN include prenatal healthcare, early childhood healthcare, perinatal coaching that strengthens early attachment between parents and their children, home visits that provide support, education, and community linkages for new parents, and support programs for children with special health and developmental problems. Physicians, nurses, emergency medical technicians and other medical personnel may identify and report suspected cases of CAN, provide diagnostic and treatment services, provide expert testimony in child protection judicial proceedings, provide information to parents regarding the needs, care and treatment of children, identify and provide support for families at risk of CAN, develop and conduct primary prevention programs, provide training on medical aspects of CAN, and participate in multidisciplinary CAN prevention teams.

However, prevention of CAN is not the sole responsibility of any single professional group, but a shared community concern. National plans of action need to be developed in collaboration with all relevant governmental and non-governmental agencies in order to jointly develop priorities and objectives, define one another's responsibilities and work together. Plans should include review and reform of legislation and policy, building data collection and research capacity, strengthening services for victims, and developing and assessing prevention responses. National plans may be modeled on the *Guide to UN Resources and Activities for the Prevention of Interpersonal Violence,*[35] and should concentrate on evidence-based interventions.[36] Available empirical evidence supports the efficacy of early childhood interventions, such as home visits, in reducing CAN. Other interventions with promising results include parenting and family therapy, life-skills and social competency programs, treatment for mental disorders, cognitive behavioral therapy and early detection of at-risk families. Many Arab countries have developed child protection services, usually in the form of child or family protection units, but it seems that only Syria has developed a comprehensive national child protection plan.[37]

References

1 Krug E, Dahlberg L, Mercy J *et al. World Report on Violence and Health.* Geneva: World Health Organization; 2002.
2 World Health Assembly. *Prevention of Violence: public health priority.* Geneva: World Health Organization, 1996.

3 Dubowitz H, DePanfilis D. *Handbook for Child Protection Practice.* Thousand Oaks, CA: Sage; 2000.

4 United States Department of Health and Human Services, Administration on Children, Youth and Families. *Child Maltreatment 2000.* Washington, DC: US Government Printing Office; 2002.

5 Finkelhor D. The international epidemiology of child sexual abuse. *Child Abuse Negl* 1994; **18 (5):** 409–17.

6 Al-Mahroos FT. Child abuse and neglect in the Arab Peninsula. *Saudi Med J* 2007; **28 (2):** 241–8.

7 *Proceedings: symposium on child protection.* Damascus, Syria: Rainbow for a Better Childhood; 2004.

8 Haj-Yahia MM, Tamish S. The rates of child sexual abuse and its psychological consequences as revealed by a study among Palestinian university students. *Child Abuse Negl* 2001; **25 (10):** 1303–27.

9 Jumaian A. Prevalence and long-term impact of child sexual abuse among a sample of male college students in Jordan. *East Mediterr Health J* 2001; **7 (3):** 435–40.

10 *Proceedings: MENA [Middle Eastern and North African] regional consultation on violence against children.* Cairo, Egypt: National Council of Childhood and Motherhood; 2005.

11 Shalhoub-Kevorkian N. Disclosure of child abuse in conflict areas. *Violence Against Women* 2005; **11 (10):** 1263–91.

12 Cicchetti D, Carlson V. *Child Maltreatment: theory and research on the causes and consequences of child abuse and neglect.* New York, NY: Cambridge University Press; 1989.

13 Coohey C, Braun N. Toward an integrated framework for understanding child physical abuse. *Child Abuse Negl* 1997; **21:** 1081–94.

14 Schilling EA, Aseltine RH, Jr, Gore S. Adverse childhood experiences and mental health in young adults: a longitudinal survey. *BMC Public Health* 2007; **7:** 30.

15 Perry BD, Pollard R, Blakely T *et al.* Childhood trauma, the neurobiology of adaptation and "use-dependent" development of the brain: How "states" become "traits". *Inf Mental Health J* 1995; **16:** 271–91.

16 Willis DJ, Holden EW, Rosenberg M. *Prevention of Child Maltreatment: developmental and ecological perspectives.* New York, NY: John Wiley & Sons; 1992.

17 Heide KM, Solomon EP. Biology, childhood trauma, and murder: rethinking justice. *Int J Law Psychiatry* 2006; **29 (3):** 220–33.

18 Egeland B, Sroufe LA. Attachment and early maltreatment. *Child Development* 1981; **52:** 44–52.

19 Alreshoud A. *Child Abuse and Neglect Among Delinquents in Saudi Arabia.* Pittsburgh: University of Pittsburgh; 1997.

20 McCrae JS, Chapman MV, Christ SL. Profile of children investigated for sexual abuse: association with psychopathology symptoms and services. *Am J Orthopsychiatry* 2006; **76 (4):** 468–81.

21 Paolucci EO, Genuis ML, Violato C. A meta-analysis of the published research on the effects of child sexual abuse. *J Psychol* 2001; **135:** 17–36.

22 Block RW, Krebs NF. Failure to thrive as a manifestation of child neglect. *Pediatrics* 2005; **116:** 1234–7.

23 Ahmed HJ, Ilardi I, Antognoli A *et al.* An epidemic of *Neisseria gonorrhoeae* in a Somali orphanage. *Int J STD AIDS* 1992; **3 (1):** 52–3.

24 Felitti VJ, Anda RF, Nordenberg D *et al.* Relationship of childhood abuse and

household dysfunction to many of the leading causes of death in adults. *Am J Prev Med* 1998; **14:** 245–58.

25 Bappal B, George M, Nair R *et al.* Factitious hypoglycemia: a tale from the Arab world. *Pediatrics* 2001; **107 (1):** 180–1.

26 Berg B, Jones DP. Outcome of psychiatric intervention in factitious illness by proxy (Munchausen's syndrome by proxy). *Arch Dis Child* 1999; **81:** 465–72.

27 Rubin DM, Christian CW, Bilaniuk LT. Occult head injury in high-risk abused children. *Pediatrics* 2003; **111:** 1382–6.

28 Sugar NF, Taylor JA, Feldman KW. Bruises in infants and toddlers: those who don't cruise rarely bruise. *Arch Pediatr Adolesc Med* 1999; **153:** 399–403.

29 Kocher MS, Kasser JR. Orthopaedic aspects of child abuse. *J Am Acad Orthop Surg* 2000; **8 (1):** 10–20.

30 Adams JA, Harper K, Knudson S *et al.* Examination findings in legally confirmed child sexual abuse: it's normal to be normal. *Pediatrics* 1994; **94:** 310–17.

31 Christopher NC, Anderson D, Gaertner L *et al.* Childhood injuries and the importance of documentation in the emergency department. *Pediatr Emerg Care* 1995; **11:** 52–7.

32 Conway EE. Nonaccidental head injury in infants: the shaken baby syndrome revisited. *Pediatric Annals* 1998; **27:** 677–90.

33 Belfer RA, Klein BL, Orr L. Use of the skeletal survey in the evaluation of child maltreatment. *Am J Emerg Med* 2001; **19 (2):** 122–4.

34 Lonergan GJ, Baker AM, Morey MK *et al.* From the archives of the AFIP. Child abuse: radiologic-pathologic correlation. *Radiographics* 2003; **23:** 811–45.

35 Anon. *Guide to United Nations Resources and Activities for the Prevention of Interpersonal Violence.* 2002 [cited 2007, 3 May]. Available from: www.who.int/violence_injury_ prevention/media/en/633pdf

36 Kluger MP, Alexander G, Curtis PA. *What Works in Child Welfare.* Washington, DC: CWLA Press; 2000.

37 Commission for Family Affairs. *National Child Protection Plan.* Damascus, Syria: UNICEF; 005.

CHAPTER 7

Domestic conflict and violence

(* *Aisha Hamdan*

Introduction

Violence against women is a widespread global phenomenon that physically, psychologically and sexually damages victims. It extends across boundaries of class, education, income, ethnicity, culture and age. No society is free of this type of violence; there is only variation in the patterns and trends that exist in different countries.[1]

Domestic violence is the most prevalent form of violence against women. A World Health Organization (WHO) multi-country study of over 24000 women in 10 countries reported that between 15% and 71% of women had experienced physical or sexual violence by an intimate partner in their lifetime, with most sites ranging from 30% to 60%. Women in Japan were least likely to have experienced physical or sexual violence, while the greatest amount of violence was reported by women living in Bangladesh, Ethiopia, Peru and the United States.[2]

The range for current violence (one or more acts within the past year) was between 3% (Serbia and Montenegro) and 54% (Ethiopia), with most sites falling between 20% and 33%.[2] The majority of women who had been physically abused experienced more than one incident of violence. Between 20% and 75% had experienced one or more acts of emotional abuse (being insulted, humiliated, intimidated or scared on purpose, or being threatened).[2]

Research seems to suggest that the prevalence of domestic violence in the Arab region is similar to that reported in other areas of the world. The differences seem to rest on the cultural underpinnings of violence against women, lack of identification, barriers to change, and the challenge of identifying appropriate intervention techniques. This chapter will address some of those issues as well as provide culturally appropriate suggestions for screening and intervention, primarily geared toward primary healthcare providers.

Definitions of violence against women and domestic violence

The United Nations *Declaration on the Elimination of Violence Against Women* defines violence against women as "any act of gender-based violence that results in, or is likely to result in, physical, sexual or psychological harm or suffering to women, including threats of such acts, coercion or arbitrary deprivation of liberty, whether occurring in public or in private life".[3] The *Declaration* defines violence against women within three realms: violence occurring within the family (battering, sexual abuse of children, female genital cutting and other traditional practices harmful to women); within the general community (rape, sexual abuse, sexual harassment, trafficking in women, forced prostitution); and violence perpetrated or condoned by the State.[3]

As defined by the United Nations Children's Fund (UNICEF), domestic violence includes violence perpetrated by intimate partners or other family members, and manifested through:

- *physical abuse* such as slapping, beating, arm twisting, stabbing, strangling, burning, choking, kicking, threats with an object or weapon, and murder. It also includes such traditional practices as female genital cutting and wife inheritance
- *psychological abuse* which includes behavior that is intended to intimidate and persecute in the form of threats of abandonment or abuse, confinement to the home, surveillance, threats to take away children, destruction of objects, isolation, verbal aggression and constant humiliation
- *sexual abuse* such as coerced sex through threats, intimidation or physical force, forcing unwanted sexual acts or forcing sex with others
- *economic abuse* such as denial of funds, refusal to contribute financially, denial of food and basic needs, and controlling access to healthcare, employment etc.[1]

Effects of violence upon women's health

Domestic violence is a major cause of illness, injury and death. Physical injuries are often multiple and may include bruises, cuts, broken bones, burns and wounds. In addition to the immediate concerns related to these types of injuries, there are often long-term consequences such as scars, joint damage, loss of hearing and vision, chronic pain and physical disabilities.[4-8] Injuries caused by domestic abuse can also be fatal. It is estimated that 25% of the homicides that occur in the United States are husband–wife killings.[9] Rape and domestic violence lead to the loss of more healthy years of life for women aged 15 to 44 than do breast cancer, cervical cancer, obstructed labor, war or motor vehicle accidents.[10]

In the WHO multi-country study, women who had experienced domestic violence were significantly more likely to report poor health or very poor health than women who had never experienced violence. Abused women were also more likely to have had problems walking, completing daily activities, pain, memory loss, and dizziness. The research suggests that the physical effects of violence may last a long time after the actual incident and increase women's risk of poor health in the future.[2]

Domestic abuse also has a negative impact upon the mental health of victims and is associated with higher rates of depression, anxiety, stress-related illness, self-harm and suicide.[7,11,12] Research in the Arab world has found that violence against women results in serious psychological consequences. The more psychological, physical and sexual abuse women suffered, the more likely they were to be distressed, angry and fearful; to experience higher levels of depression, anxiety and stress; and to have lower self-esteem.[13,14]

Prevalence in Arab countries

There is a lack of statistical and official data on the prevalence of domestic violence in the Arab region, mainly due to the sensitive nature of the subject.[15] Existing surveys may underestimate the extent of the problem due to underreporting. The research that has been done thus far suggests that the rate of domestic violence is as common in Arab society as it is in other parts of the world. The following section surveys some of the results of research in this region.

A Demographic and Health Survey conducted among a national random sample of 14 779 women in Egypt found that one out of three women had been beaten at least once since marriage. Of this group about 45% had been beaten at least once over the previous year, and one-third of those were abused during pregnancy. Of those who had been beaten, 18% said that they had been hurt as a result of the beating, and 10% mentioned that they required medical attention.[16]

Haj-Yahia conducted two national surveys in the West Bank and Gaza strip of Palestine using systematic random samples of 2410 and 1334 respectively.[17] The results showed that about 52% of women participating in the first survey and 54% of women in the second survey reported that they had experienced one or more acts of physical violence at least once during the 12 months prior to the study.[17] In the first survey, approximately 23%, 33.6% and 34.3% of the women indicated that they had experienced mild, moderate or severe psychological abuse, respectively, by their spouses. Similar results (21.5%, 32% and 33.7%) were obtained in the second survey. Examples of psychological abuse included insulting, cursing, using abusive language, name-calling, controlling, reprimanding, belittling thoughts, beliefs and attitudes.[17]

A study conducted in Syria of 411 women randomly selected from primary care centers found that current physical abuse (battering at least three times during the previous year) was present in 23% of those investigated and among 26% of married women. Regular abuse (battering at least once weekly) was found in 3.3% of married women.[18]

In a study of domestic violence in the Palestinian refugee camps of Jordan, women were asked if they had experienced specific acts of violence, while men were asked if they had carried out these acts against their wives. The prevalence rate of lifetime beating was found to be 44.7%, with men reporting a higher prevalence rate (48.9%) than women (42.5%). Slapping was the most common beating behavior (36%), followed by pushing, grabbing or shoving (23.5%), and other unspecified acts of violence (22.9%). Nineteen percent of women reported having being beaten during the past year and 13.7% of men reported that they had beaten their wives during the same period.[19]

The results of a study in Sudan indicated that 49.6% of women reported having been victims of abuse (including assaults, threat or intimidation). Approximately 20% of the women had experienced physical violence. Thirty percent had been threatened with physical injury. The typical violent episode in this study involved a combination of assault, threats and verbal abuse.[20]

Dynamics in the Arab context

While the prevalence and types of abuse that occur in Arab society may be commensurate with those in other parts of the world, there are unique cultural dynamics that need to be taken into consideration. These dynamics, including structure, values and features, provide a context within which to understand the persistence of domestic violence within Arab families and the challenges posed for intervention.

Family unity, privacy and honor

In Arab society, the family is considered to be a fundamental social institution whose unity and cohesiveness must be maintained.[21] It is central to the individual's social identity and economic status.[22] This often leads members to forego personal needs and desires in exchange for the well-being of the family and to maintain the family's reputation and honor.[21]

There is a tendency in the Arab world to view domestic violence as a private family matter rather than a problem that requires the intervention of social welfare and social control agents.[17,23-5] In a study by Haj-Yahia, 80% of the men and women indicated that wife abuse "doesn't justify reporting the husband to the legal authorities".[25] Emphasis is placed upon family privacy, reputation and solidarity. There is a fear that acknowledging domestic violence as a problem that requires intervention will violate family boundaries and harm the reputation and honor of the family. This could result in social, economic and educational consequences for all family members.[23] Women themselves may feel reluctance to seek help due to the shame, perceived or otherwise, that may fall on her and her family. It is expected that individuals will sacrifice their own needs and welfare for the sake of the family unit.[21,23]

Gender roles

Traditional Arab social and family structure is patriarchal and characterized by male authority and control. As head of the household, men are expected to maintain family honor and cohesion based upon loyalties to parents, siblings and spouse.[26] Families generally function with clearly defined gender and marital roles. Husbands are responsible for providing financial support for family members, making important decisions, and disciplining when family honor or status is threatened.[26] Women are generally dependent upon their husbands, are submissive and obedient, and are responsible for the children and household.

Some theorists suggest that men who believe their power or position is being threatened may resort to violence in order to restore their dominance. They may also have been taught that violence is an acceptable method of solving problems and conflicts as well as a way to maintain authority and power.[21] A woman who fails to fulfill her traditional role appropriately may be at risk of physical or emotional abuse (*see* discussion below).

Haj-Yahia argues that the ultimate cause of wife abuse and battering is sexism, gender inequality, and gender-role stereotypes characterized by the domination of men over women within a patriarchal society.[27] At the same time, however, he cites an extensive meta-analytic review of studies conducted in Western societies that refutes his hypothesis. This review found limited support for the hypothesis that "predicted that maritally violent men, in contrast to maritally nonviolent men, would report more positive attitudes toward use of marital violence, more conservative gender attitudes, and a more traditional masculine schema".[27,30]

This evidence supports the notion that there is nothing inherently wrong with the cultural structure of patriarchy. This conclusion is further supported by the fact that domestic violence happens in all cultures, even those in which "gender equality" is heavily promoted. The greater likelihood is that there are other intervening variables that contribute to the occurrence of domestic violence. Some of these possible variables are discussed below.

Justifications for abuse and blaming the victim

Societies have different perceptions of wife abuse and attitudes toward the victims and perpetrators. These differences are reflected in cultural perceptions of justifications for abuse, tolerance and leniency toward violent husbands, and blaming wives for violence against them.[21] Within Arab society, research seems to indicate that domestic abuse is justified for various reasons and blame is often placed upon the victim.

Haj-Yahia reported that 28% of Arab men in his study strongly agreed or agreed that "sometimes it is OK for a man to beat his wife".[27] Between 15% and

62% strongly agreed or agreed that wife-beating is justified for certain reasons. The strongest justification involved unfaithful sexual behavior (62% strongly agreed or agreed that "a sexually unfaithful wife deserves to be beaten"). Other justifications included insulting the husband in front of his friends; constantly disobeying the husband; disrespect for his parents, siblings or other relatives; and lying to the husband. Older and less educated men showed a greater tendency to justify wife-beating.[27]

Earlier studies by Haj-Yahia reported similar results, in that between 23% and 71% of men and between 14% and 69% of women expressed support for wife-beating for certain reasons.[24,25] The reasons included those mentioned above as well as challenging the husband's manhood, refusing to be intimate with the husband, failing to meet the husband's expectations, and reminding the husband of his weak points.[24,25] Eighty percent of women surveyed in rural Egypt said that beatings were common and often justified, particularly if the woman refused to have intimate relations with her husband.[16]

These findings contrast with those reported in studies conducted in the United States and Australia. One study in the United States found that 18.8% of women accepted the idea of situations in which beatings are justified, with over 20% blaming the victim for her beatings.[28] Similar results were obtained in a study from Australia, in which 20% of the respondents believed that wife assault was justified under certain conditions.[29] It is interesting to note that the WHO multi-country study found that substantially more women accept wife abuse in the case of infidelity (actual or suspected) than for any other reason. It is also frequently tolerated in situations where women disobey their spouses.[2]

Related to justifications for abuse, Arab men tend to blame the wife for violence inflicted upon her. In the study reported by Haj-Yahia, 33% of husbands in the study strongly agreed or agreed that "in most cases, the wife is responsible for violence against her, due to her mistaken behavior".[27] Cases in which blaming was considered most warranted included those in which the wife "treats her husband inappropriately" and "takes care of her children inadequately". Older and less educated men had a greater tendency to blame women for the violence.[27] Blaming the wife was correlated with less propensity to hold violent husbands responsible for their behavior, justifying the behavior due to personal and life conditions of the husband. These results are similar to those obtained in earlier studies by Haj-Yahia.[24,25]

Predisposing or precipitating factors

While research in the area is nascent, the work that has been completed suggests possible predisposing or precipitating factors related to domestic violence. Correlational studies have looked mainly at socio-demographic factors such as socioeconomic status, place of residence, and level of education. Other studies have focused on triggers or precipitating factors. It should be noted that these results are not so different from those obtained in other parts of the world.

Socio-demographic factors

In two national surveys conducted in Palestinian society, Haj-Yahia (2000) found that the most significant socio-demographic predictors of abuse and battering were: place of residence (rural areas and refugee camps more than urban areas), husbands with a low level of education, low family income, women who do not work for a salary, wives whose level of education is higher than that of their husband, and religion (Muslim women more than Christian women).[17] Further analyses revealed that Muslim women compared with Christian women are less educated, more likely not to work for a salary, come from low-income families with serious economic problems, have more children, and live in refugee camps and rural areas. Rural and refugee families are large, live in difficult conditions, and experience serious economic hardship.[17] These results suggest the need for future research investigating the role of family resources and family stress in precipitating and/or exacerbating domestic violence. This approach is validated by research from the United States indicating that although abuse occurs in all economic groups, women in the low-income group are four times as likely to be victims of violence committed by an intimate partner or male relative.[31]

Research conducted in Syria found that married women are more likely to be physically abused than single, divorced or widowed women.[18] Husbands are the most common perpetrators of the abuse. Women living in rural areas and those with lower socioeconomic status are more likely to be abused. Abused women tend to be less educated, with less-educated husbands. They also tend to marry and start motherhood at an earlier age.[18]

A study of women attending a medical centre in Sudan found that abused women in comparison to a control group were younger, of lower education status, unemployed, and had been married a shorter time. Abusive husbands were less educated, less likely to be employed, and were more likely to be alcohol or drug abusers.[20]

Several of these studies, as well as many conducted in other parts of the world, have found a connection between lower socioeconomic status and domestic violence (although it does occur in all levels).[20,32] Poverty, and the associated feelings of hopelessness and crowding, can result in increased conflicts in relationships. It can also lead to frustration among men in a culture that emphasizes their role as providers to the household.[20] Unemployment and the stress of searching for work increase the risk that a husband will abuse his wife. In a study by Ahmed and Elmardi, 40% of the husbands of abused women were unemployed compared to 10% of the husbands in the control group.[20]

The increase in female employment may also contribute to tensions within the marital relationship. In conservative Arab society, a situation where the wife is working and the husband is unemployed represents a reversal of cultural norms and may generate family conflict.[20]

Triggers

A qualitative study of factors related to domestic violence in Lebanese families identified three main categories of triggers for abuse: unmet marital role expectations, conflict with in-laws, and substance abuse.[26] In the category of unmet role expectations, some specific examples of precipitants included failure to fulfill basic domestic responsibilities, childcare issues, the husband's inability to provide for the family at a standard set by the wife (and subsequent demands of the wife), disobedience, and lack of deference to the husband's decisions.[26] Interpersonal stress between a husband's mother and wife was common. This was often combined with the husband's struggle with conflicting loyalties. In general, couples who lived on their own were less likely to experience abuse problems. Substance abuse was noted in a small proportion of the sample.[26]

In a study from Sudan, immediate provoking events for violence included suspicion of illicit relations, talking back, not obeying the husband, not having food prepared on time, refusing sexual relations, failure to care for the home or children adequately, going out of the home without permission and questioning the husband about his money or illicit relations.[20]

Options available for victims of domestic violence

Four strategies used by abused women to cope with violence have been reported in the literature:
1 personal strategies (e.g. placating the husband, avoiding contact with him, physically resisting violence by attacking back)
2 seeking help from informal or semi-formal agents (e.g. family members and relatives, friends, neighbors, and informal organizations in the community)
3 seeking help from formal agents (e.g. police, courts, social services)
4 leaving the abusive husband (either separation or divorce).[33]

In the West, women may be more likely to pursue the third and fourth options above, while women in Arab countries are more likely to resort to the first and second. For various reasons, the options available to victims of domestic violence in Arab countries are more limited than those in the West. Overall, there is a shortage of essential services for abused women. This shortage may be due to the social and cultural variables discussed earlier that emphasize the privacy of the family and explicit gender roles. Services such as hotlines, shelters and programs aimed at "empowering" women economically and socially may be considered unacceptable at a societal level due to their contradiction with social norms.

Mental health services can be stigmatizing as well, particularly for women. The utilization of such services could affect marital prospects and increase the possibility of separation or divorce.[22] Stigma may be reduced by integrating mental health services into non-threatening settings such as primary care clinics.[22]

Cultural norms restrict victims from seeking legal assistance or medical attention. As previously mentioned, there is a tendency to view wife abuse as a personal and family problem that should be dealt with inside the family without intervention from social service agencies or the law.[34] In a study of Jordanian women, 62.9% and 83.7% of the participants strongly agreed or agreed that "If I heard a woman being attacked by her husband, it would be best to do nothing", and "a battered woman should be given all of the needed help and support by her family", respectively.[34]

In Arab society, divorce is socially intolerable, particularly when requested by the wife. Divorce is difficult to obtain and the process can be complicated.[20] If a woman does obtain a divorce, she may experience social isolation and even violence from other family members.[20] There may also be concerns about the children as custody may go to the father. Husbands whose wives ask for a divorce may be threatened with being unable to see their children.[15]

Women who are poorly educated and unskilled have limited access to employment. Therefore they lack financial support unless family members are willing to provide it.[20] A woman may receive temporary protection, shelter and support from her family of origin, but she is expected to remain loyal to her husband and his family. She may be pressured to return to her husband in order to maintain the unity of the family and the reputation of their family of origin, as well as to honor her commitment to her husband and children.[21]

Abused women are reluctant to report domestic violence to legal authorities due to the risk of facing social isolation and ostracism. Women who use the law to remove husbands from the home or issue a protection order against them may be blamed for weakening family unity and stability.[21,23,34] Resorting to legal measures may also become a source of danger for the wife rather than a means to protect her.

Arab society views the law as a punitive measure against the husband rather than a protective or deterrent measure.[21] For these reasons, violent husbands are rarely brought to court or faced with other legal sanctions.[34] In the majority of cases, police, health professionals, and other services are of limited assistance.

Research seems to suggest that any initiative-taking on the wife's part may actually lead to an escalation of violence.[26] Passive resignation, on the other hand, is linked to the process of ongoing physical abuse.[26] A less direct but effective method involves participation from extended family members and community networks. This option allows both partners to maintain cultural expectations while keeping the family intact.[26]

Screening for domestic violence

Domestic violence often goes unrecognized in medical practice.[35] Women rarely disclose information of this nature unless they are directly asked.[36] Barriers to screening include a lack of clinical guidelines, brevity of medical visits, clinicians' discomfort with the topic, and misconceptions about the typical victims of abuse.[37-9] For patients, past failures with the medical system; embarrassment, shame, or guilt about the abuse; cultural and language barriers; and fear of reprisal contribute to lack of disclosure about abuse[17,38] These factors are likely to be exacerbated due to the cultural context and subsequent concerns related to maintaining family status and honor.

Physicians should make it a routine practice to ask patients about physical abuse, due to its high prevalence and significant impact on the health status of women.[40-2] History-taking and interview should include at least one or two questions related to domestic violence. If necessary, more detailed information should be obtained in a non-threatening and delicate manner. Research has found that the simple inclusion of one or two questions about domestic abuse during the patient interview can significantly improve the rates of recognition.[43-6] These questions may include the following: "Do you ever feel unsafe at home?", "Has anyone at home hit you or tried to injure you in any way?", "Have you ever felt afraid of your spouse?"[37] The interviewer should introduce the topic in a non-threatening manner by saying, for example, "We're concerned about the health effects of domestic abuse, so we routinely ask our patients a few questions."[37]

It is clearly advisable that screening of patients be carried out in private. While confidentiality is important in any case, it is particularly significant in this environment due to the risks of retaliation by the abuser and other negative consequences. A woman should never be questioned about domestic violence in the presence of her spouse.[37] Studies from the Arab world have suggested that women are willing to disclose abuse issues when questioned in a supportive manner with assurances of strict confidentiality.[20]

Appropriate interventions in social and cultural context

In general, during intervention, it is important to maintain the essential values of the community while attempting to effect change. Attempts to cope with the problem both within and outside of the family should emphasize privacy and discretion. Importance should be placed on preserving family unity and the reputation of the nuclear family and families of origin. Some middle ground should be found between opposing violence and assisting the wife in understanding and supporting her husband.[21]

Within our society, the family is an important focus of life and daily interactions, reflecting its collective nature. For this reason, prevention or intervention efforts should consider the context of the nuclear and extended family.[22] One study of this issue found that 92% of women indicated that coping with violence should begin with the nuclear family. Approximately 77% indicated that they would also recommend involving the families of origin and extended families in certain situations. Only 15% indicated that they would recommend seeking help from social services or reporting to the police in extremely difficult cases.[21]

The group or family may provide the individual with protection and security, as well as emotional and practical support during times of crises. Family members may be involved in the resolution of issues as well as in the actual process of helping.[22] They should be educated about the incidence of abuse and violence and the physical and mental health consequences of such behaviors as well as the importance of supporting and protecting abused women.[13] Care must be taken throughout the process to avoid challenging the hierarchies or role patterns within the family since this may lead to alienation.[22]

It may also be beneficial to focus on ways in which the wife may change her own behavior toward her husband as a way to prevent violence. This reflects the cultural tendency to expect that the wife will change her behavior toward her husband and assume responsibility for changing his violent behavior.[33] In a study of women's patterns of coping with wife abuse it was found that women preferred the following patterns of coping:

1   the wife tries to persuade her husband to change
2   the wife changes her own behavior toward her husband
3   the wife tries to appease her husband and encourage intimacy
4   the wife stays away from her husband when he is angry
5   the wife seeks advice from welfare services on ways to improve her behavior toward her husband.[33]

In the same study, a moderate level of support was found for the following coping patterns:

1   the wife seeks help from welfare agencies to persuade the abusive husband to receive treatment
2   the wife asks a clergyman or well-known community figure to intervene
3   the wife requests assistance and support from her parents and brothers.

Strong opposition to the following coping patterns was found:

1   threatening the husband with a request for a divorce
2   going to a battered women's shelter
3   filing for divorce in court
4   attacking the husband in the way he attacked her
5   filing a complaint against the husband with the police
6   leaving home without telling the husband her whereabouts.[33]

The goals of intervention with abused women should focus on physical and psychological health and safety. Haj-Yahia suggests that human service intervention should involve:

- routine screening and identification of domestic violence
- validation of the experiences
- considerations of the responses to trauma and psychological consequences in assessment and intervention planning
- safety planning with victims
- record-keeping, documentation and dissemination
- direct interventions with abused women.[13,24]

This requires an interdisciplinary approach with health, mental health and human service practitioners, relevant community leaders and significant members of the women's extended families or other networks.[13]

Approaches for the primary care provider

The primary care provider should screen patients for a history of abuse, identify relevant historical and physical findings, document the findings in the medical record, refer patients for appropriate services, and assess whether the patient is in immediate danger.[37] If a patient reveals abuse, the provider should ask about the nature of the abuse; the date, time and circumstances of the event; previous incidents; and resultant injuries.[37] Assessment should also focus on the victim's strategies and skills for coping with the situation and the availability of formal and informal resources. It is also important to determine the extent to which family members are willing to assist in deterring violent behavior of the husband.[21]

Given the patriarchal quality of Arab society, patients often place a significant amount of responsibility on practitioners to provide solutions to their problems with little contribution from the patient themselves. Practitioners are seen as authority figures whose advice should be followed without confrontation. For this reason, helping should be direct and clear with specific goals. Guidance, explanations and instructions should be provided.[22]

The primary care provider could also facilitate a mediation process, which is a solid structure within the Arab milieu. Suggestions may be offered to the patient to bring in a relative who is a trusted confidant. This person could begin the process of mediation and help to identify allies and coalitions that the patient can draw upon for support. Taking advantage of such a well established tradition may enhance the likelihood of a successful outcome.

Conclusion

Domestic violence is a major contributor to the poor health of women around the world. There is increasing awareness that it is a significant health problem as well as a risk factor for other diseases and conditions. Professionals within the health sector have the potential to play an important role in breaking the cycle of violence against women.[2] This can be achieved through appropriate prevention, identification and intervention strategies, particularly taking into consideration cultural and social factors.

Research indicates that the prevalence of domestic violence in the Arab region is similar to that in other areas of the world. Practitioners who work with this population should be sensitive to the context in which abuse occurs and make use of resources within the victim's environment to her advantage.[33] Due to the complexity of the issue, future research on domestic violence in the Arab world should take an integrated approach and consider intrapersonal, interpersonal, familial, socio-cultural, structural, political and sociolegal constructs.[27]

References

1 United Nations Children's Fund. *Domestic Violence Against Women and Girls.* Florence, Italy: UNICEF Innocenti Research Centre; 2000.

2 World Health Organization. *WHO Multi-country Study on Women's Health and Domestic Violence Against Women.* Geneva, Switzerland: WHO; 2005. Available at: http://www.who.int/gender/violence/who_multicountry_study/en/. Accessed 26 December 2006.

3 United Nations. *Declaration on the Elimination of Violence Against Women.* December 20, 1993. Available from: http://www.un.org/documents/ga/res/48/a48r104.htm. Accessed 24 December 2006.

4 Abbott J. Injuries and illnesses of domestic violence. *Ann Emerg Med* 1997; **29:** 781–5.

5 Council of Scientific Affairs. Violence against women: relevance for medical practioners. *JAMA* 1992; **267:** 3184–9.

6 Muelleman RL, Lenaghan PA, Pakieser RA. Battered women: injury locations and types. *Ann Emerg Med* 1996; **28:** 486–92.

7 Peckover S. Domestic abuse and women's health: the challenge of primary care. *Prim Health Care Res Dev* 2002; **3:** 151–8.

8 Plichta S. The effect of woman abuse on health care utilisation and health status: a literature review. *Women's Health Issues* 1992; **2:** 154–63.

9 United States Department of Justice. *Criminal Victimization in the US: national crime report.* Washington, DC: Government Printing Office; 1995.

10 World Bank. *World Development Report;* 1993.

11 Andrews B, Brown GW. Marital violence in the community: a biographical approach. *Br J Psychiatry* 1988; **153:** 305–12.

12 Jaffe P, Wolfe DA, Wilson S *et al.* Emotional and physical health problems of battered women. *Can J of Psychiatry* 1986; **31:** 625–9.

13 Haj-Yahia MM. Wife abuse and its psychological consequences as revealed by the first Palestinian National Survey on Violence Against Women. *J Fam Psychol* 1999; **13 (4):** 642–62.

14 Haj-Yahia MM. Implications of wife-abuse and battering for self-esteem, depression and anxiety as revealed by the second Palestinian National Survey on Violence Against Women. *J Fam Iss* 2000a; **21 (4):** 435–63.

15 Almosaed N. Violence against women: a cross-cultural perspective. *J Muslim Affairs* 2004; **24 (1):** 67–88.

16 El-Zanaty F, Hussein EM, Shawky GA *et al. Egypt Demographic and Health Survey 1995.* Cairo, Egypt: National Population Council; 1996.

17 Haj-Yahia MM. The incidence of wife abuse and battering and some sociodemographic correlates as revealed by two national surveys in Palestinian society. *J Fam Violence* 2000b; **15 (4):** 347–74.

18 Maziak W, Asfar T. Physical abuse in low-income women in Aleppo, Syria. *Health Care for Women Int* 2003; **24:** 313–26.

19 Khawaja M, Barazi R. Prevalence of wife beating in Jordanian refugee camps: reports by men and women. *J Epidemiol Community Health* 2005; **59:** 840–1.

20 Ahmed AM, Elmardi, AE. A study of domestic violence among women attending a medical centre in Sudan. *East Mediterr Health J* 2005; **11 (1–2):** 164–74.

21 Haj-Yahia MM. Wife abuse and battering in the sociocultural context of Arab society. *Fam Process* 2000c; **39 (2):** 237–55.

22 Al-Krenawi A, Graham JR. *Culturally Sensitive Social Work Practice with Arab Clients in Mental Health Settings*; 2000. Available at: http://www.socialworkers.org/pressroon/events/911/alkrenawi.asp. Accessed 5 December 2006.

23 Douki S, Nacef F, Belhadj A *et al.* Violence against women in Arab and Islamic countries. *Arch Women's Ment Health* 2003; **6:** 165–71.

24 Haj-Yahia MM. A patriarchal perspective on beliefs about wife-beating among Arab Palestinian men from the West Bank and Gaza strip. *J Fam Issues* 1998a; **19:** 595–621.

25 Haj-Yahia MM. Beliefs about wife-beating among Palestinian women: the influence of patriarchal ideology. *Violence Against Women* 1998b; **4:** 533–58.

26 Kenaan CK, El-Hadad A, Balian, SA. Factors associated with domestic violence in low-income Lebanese families. *J Nurs Scholarsh* 1998; **30 (4):** 357–62.

27 Haj-Yahia MM. Beliefs about wife-beating among Arab men from Israel: the influence of their patriarchal ideology. *J Fam Violence* 2003; **18 (4):** 193–206.

28 Gentemann K. Wife beating: attitudes of non-clinical population. *Victimology* 1984; **9:** 109–19.

29 Mugford J, Mugford S, Easteal P. Social justice, public perceptions, and spouse assault in Australia. *Soc Justice* 1989; **16:** 103.

30 Sugarman DB, Frankel SL. Patriarchal ideology and wife assaults: a meta-analytic review. *J Fam Violence* 1996; **11 (1):** 13–40.

31 Centers for Diseases Control. *DHHS Annual "Health, United States" Report, with Special Profile of Women's Health.* Atlanta, GA: CDC; 1996.

32 Kyriacou DN *et al.* Risk factors for injury to women from domestic violence against women. *New Engl J Med* 1999; **341 (25):** 1892–8.

33 Haj-Yahia MM. Attitudes of Arab women toward different patterns of coping with wife abuse. *J Interpers Violence* 2002a; **17 (7):** 721–45.

34 Haj-Yahia MM. Beliefs of Jordanian women about wife-beating. *Psychol J Women Quarterly* 2002b; **26:** 282–91.

35 Reid SA, Glasser M. Primary care physicians recognition of and attitudes toward domestic violence. *Acad Med* 1997; **72 (1):** 51–3.

36 Leserman J, Drossman, DA. Sexual and physical abuse history and medical practice. *Gen Hosp Psychiatry* 1995; **17 (2):** 71–4.

37 Eisenstat SA, Bancroft L. Primary care: domestic violence. *New Engl J Med* 1999; **341 (12):** 886–92.

38 Sugg NK, Inui T. Primary care physicians' response to domestic violence: opening Pandora's box. *JAMA* 1992; **267:** 3157–60.

39 Cohen S, De Vos E, Newberger E. Barriers to physician identification and treatment of family violence: lessons from five communities. *Acad Med* 1997; **72: Suppl:** S19–S25.

40 Alpert EJ. Violence in intimate relationships and the practicing internist: new "disease" or new agenda? *Ann Intern Med* 1995; **123 (10):** 774–81.

41 Warshaw C. Intimate partner abuse: developing a framework for change in medical education. *Acad Med* 1997; **72 (1 Suppl):** S26–S37.

42 Warshaw C, Alpert E. Integrating routine inquiry about domestic violence into daily practice. *Ann Intern Med* 1999; **131 (8):** 619–20.

43 Freund KM, Bak SM, Blackhall L. Identifying domestic violence in primary care practice. *J Gen Intern Med* 1996; **11 (1):** 44–6.

44 Kripke EN, Steele G, O'Brien MK *et al.* Domestic violence training program for residents. *J Gen Intern Med* 1998; **13 (12):** 839–41.

45 Thompson RS, Rivara FP, Thompson DC *et al.* Identification and management of domestic violence: a randomized trial. *Am J Prev Med* 2000; **19 (4):** 253–63.

46 Feldhaus KM, Koziol-McLain J, Amsbury HL *et al.* Accuracy of 3 brief screening questions for detecting partner violence in the emergency department. *JAMA* 1997; **277:** 1357–61.

CHAPTER 8

Disability

☾★ *Arwa K Abdul-Haq*

Introduction

Disability describes a condition in which the ability of a person to perform activities that include some or all of the tasks of daily living is compromised. There are many factors that predispose individuals and populations to disabling conditions; some of these will be discussed in this chapter.

There is growing evidence regarding the association between disability and poverty; both of these conditions seem to share a number of common themes. These include poor education and living conditions, poor nutrition and lack of access to healthcare. Moreover, disability compromises the income-generating potential of families, contributing further to poverty, and resulting in a "cycle of disadvantage". In addition to economic shortcomings, disabilities are associated with social stigma that can have a devastating emotional impact on the disabled and their families. Disability seems to place a higher burden on women than men, both as victims of disability and as providers of care for the disabled.[1]

Prevalence

A new framework for defining and classifying disability is being implemented by the World Health Organization (WHO). This new classification system acknowledges that every human being can be subject to health impairment, and so may be subject to some degree of disability. The *International Classification of Functioning, Disability and Health* (ICF) draws upon a social model of disability that describes disability from the standpoint of the body, the individual and society. This classification shifts the emphasis of defining disability from the cause of the disability to a more objective measure of functional and/or social limitation. It also allows consideration of the effects that adverse or favorable environmental factors have on disability.

It is hoped that by using an objective measure of disability worldwide, its true extent and impact can be measured and studied.[2]

Because current definitions of disability vary, estimates of disability prevalence from different parts of the world are not comparable. The WHO estimates that 10% of the world population suffers from physical, sensory, intellectual or mental disability.

Developed countries tend to report higher estimates of disability than developing countries. This is likely to be due to older population structures, and better diagnostic and surveillance capabilities. Applying the 10% figure to Arab countries would result in an estimate of 30 million persons living with disability in the region.

Only very limited and incomplete data regarding the distribution of disability across gender, age and causes are available from Arab countries.

Causes of disability in the Arab world

Causes of disability in the Arab countries vary, and prevalence rates are likely to be country and region-specific. Overall, the main causes of disability are thought to be:[3]

- *motor vehicle accidents (MVA):* data on road traffic fatalities are more available and accurate than those regarding injuries and disabilities. Worldwide, MVA fatalities exceed those from malaria, TB or HIV/AIDS. The mortality per 100 000 population in the Middle East due to MVA is among the highest in the world.[4] In addition, more than half of MVA fatalities occur in people between the ages of 15 and 44, who are often breadwinners of families.[5] Also, the heaviest users of the roads include the poor.[6] If we use the mortality data as a proxy for injuries, it becomes clear that MVA are one of the major reasons for injury and disability in the region.

- *work-related injuries:* again, more accurate data are available on mortality than injuries and disabilities related to work. Obtaining data on work-related injuries is complicated by the fact that most workers, especially those in low-income brackets, are employed in the informal workforce. Rates of fatal work-related injuries in the Middle Eastern Crescent countries are reported to be between three and four times higher than those of established economies. The main factors contributing to the high accident rates are reported to be: (i) lack of an occupational safety and health culture; (ii) poor management systems; and (iii) poor supervision and enforcement of existing regulations by governments.[3,7]

- *war and military conflict:* in addition to the direct effects of violence, military conflict compromises both material and social resources, and limits access to medical and rehabilitative services, resulting in diminished ability to treat injuries and prevent disability. Unemployment and poverty resulting from conflicts exert an additional toll on the mental health of populations already terrorized by physical violence. Data from Gaza and Iraq document high rates of post-traumatic stress disorder (PTSD) and depression; both are known to compromise the productive capacity of individuals and societies.[3]

➡ *chronic and communicable diseases:* tuberculosis and malaria continue to produce considerable morbidity in some regions. HIV/AIDS rates in Arab countries remain significantly lower than in other regions.[3]

➡ *congenital and genetic diseases:* the high rates of consanguineous marriages in the Arab world result in a considerable burden of disability due to congenital and heritable genetic disorders (*see* Chapter 4, Genetic disorders). Hemoglobinopathies such as thalassemia and sickle cell anemia are prevalent in some regions, and are significant causes of morbidity and reduced earning potential.

➡ *malnutrition:* general protein and calorie malnutrition and specific vitamin and mineral deficiency syndromes such as iron deficiency anemia are common in many regions. Untreated deficiencies may result in lifelong physical and mental impairments.

Prevention of disability

Prevention efforts can be categorized into primary, secondary and tertiary strategies.

➡ *primary prevention* of disability aims at providing a safe environment and decreasing the likelihood of the occurrence of disabling injuries. This includes providing a safe work environment and the use of personal protective gear. It also includes the use of seatbelts, road safety and maintenance, and enforcement of speed limits. Improved maternal care, immunizations, nutrition programs and early childhood development programs are examples of highly effective primary prevention strategies.

➡ *secondary prevention* involves maximal treatment and rehabilitation of injuries and other conditions to prevent or decrease their potential to cause disability. This requires a strong medical and rehabilitation infrastructure.

➡ *tertiary prevention* is concerned with minimizing the negative consequences of disability through chronic management of conditions and integration into the community to enable the disabled person to lead a fulfilling life. This category includes special educational programs for the disabled.

Community attitudes

Community attitudes toward disability are important since they contribute heavily to the presence and degree of stigma associated with the condition. Changes in behavior are often observable in response to this perceived stigma.

A study from Egypt found that many individuals who suffered from profound vision loss insisted that they only had "weak eyesight" and maintained their social roles to avoid the stigma associated with disability.[8]

Although disabled children are generally accepted within families, some studies report a perceived sense of shame and rejection by the community; one survey carried out in Oman suggested that the concealment of children with disability was common.[9,10,11] It has been suggested that the presence of a handicapped child within the family may make it difficult for the child's sisters to find marriage partners in the community.[12]

A study that evaluated age-matched siblings in Lebanon found that, compared to their non-disabled sibling, individuals with disabilities were more likely to experience disadvantage in areas of education, employment, income, marital status and psychological well-being. Marital status disadvantage was most marked in lower-income groups for males, and among disabled women in all socio-economic groups.[13]

Political factors can affect perceptions toward the disabled. Negative community attitudes toward individuals suffering from disability in the Levant were historically reported to be consistent with those of surrounding regions and communities. However, after the onset of the Intifada in 1987, it is reported that in many Palestinian Christian and Muslim communities, perceptions of physical disability changed from one associated with stigma, to a more positive attitude.[1] A study from Israel that compared the responses of Jewish, Muslim and Christian adolescents suggested that the circumstances alleged to have led to disability in a hypothetical scenario (such as having been injured in military action) were the major factor determining how all three groups perceived a disabled person.[14]

Disability in children

Disability is considered one of the most important causes of vulnerability among children, especially in developing countries. Disability in children is particularly devastating because it has the potential to interfere with developmental processes and impede the acquisition of critical developmental tasks such as education, self-esteem and emotional and social development. On the other hand, this developmental plasticity may work to the individual's advantage if treatment and rehabilitation are provided in a prompt and timely manner; many potential causes of childhood disability are curable, or can be significantly ameliorated with appropriate intervention.[15,16]

A study of parental attitudes toward their disabled children among Muslim, Christian and Druze families living in Israel reported that although attitudes were generally quite positive, better educated parents tended to hold less favorable attitudes than those with less education.[17] The authors suggested that traditional attitudes toward the disabled may be more positive and inclusive than "modern" ones.

A survey carried out by the World Bank in Egypt, Jordan and Yemen estimated that between 5% and 10% of children under age 18 have at least one type of disability; many of these children face health, educational, social and psychological problems.[3] A community-based study carried out in Jeddah, Saudi Arabia, found that speech, motor or mental disabilities were most common; 60% of children with disability had one type of disability, 22% suffered from two conditions, and 19% had three or more conditions. In addition, 34% of the cases detected were the second or third child with a disability in the family.[18] Potentially modifiable maternal risk factors for having a disabled child were reported to include: early and late age of marriage and childbearing, consanguineous marriage, poor education and unemployment.[19] Another study from the United Arab Emirates (UAE) found that global developmental delay in three-year-old children was associated with a history of pregnancy complications, a family history of developmental delay, and poor maternal education.[20]

A number of studies explore stress and coping by parents (particularly mothers) of children with disabilities. Consistent with data from other countries, these studies suggest that mothers provide the major burden of caretaking of children with disabilities. Other findings, which seem more characteristic of Arab countries, include the fact that the presence of informal support (friends, family, community) is a more important factor in ameliorating maternal stress than any other single factor, including formal sources of support, such as welfare services.[21-4]

Education is one area where disabled children are most disadvantaged. Children with disabilities, particularly girls, are far more likely to be illiterate than are other groups in the region.[25] A study that measured the attitudes of university students training for teaching careers in Jordan and the UAE found that attitudes toward disabled individuals were largely negative.[26] A study of general education teachers in the UAE reported negative attitudes toward the inclusion of disabled students into general classrooms.[27]

Conclusions

People living with disability in the Arab world represent a population that has been understudied and underserved. The issue of disability has not previously received a high priority in many regions of the Arab world. In the past few years, organizations and groups have begun to work on issues such as specialized training for the disabled, sheltered work, and mainstreaming individuals with disabilities into the educational and occupational arenas.[28]

Many issues related to disability – such as the demographics and causes of disability in the region; cost-effective measures to prevent disability and improve the reach of rehabilitation programs; and assessment of community attitudes toward the disabled – all need to be researched. Understanding these features is essential in designing effective, integrated and sustainable programs and policies in the region.

References

1 Nagata K. Gender and disability in the Arab region: the challenges in the new millennium. *Asia Pacific Disability Rehabilitation Journal* 2003; **14 (1):** 10–17.

2 World Health Organization. *International Classification of Functioning, Disability and Health* [cited 2007, 16 June]. Available from: http://www.who.int/classifications/icf/en/

3 Bank W. *A Note on Disability Issues in the Middle East and North Africa.* 2005 [cited 2007, 16 June]. Available from: http://siteresources.worldbank.org/DISABILITY/Resources/Regions/MENA/MENADisabilities.doc

4 World Health Organization. *World Report on Road Traffic Injury Prevention.* 2004 [cited 2007, 16 June]. Available from: http://www.who.int/world-health-day/2004/infomaterials/world_report/chapter2.pdf

5 Kopits E, Cropper M. Traffic fatalities and economic growth. *Accid Anal Prev* 2005; **37 (1):** 169–78.

6 Ameratunga S, Hijar M, Norton R. Road-traffic injuries: confronting disparities to address a global-health problem. *Lancet* 2006; **367 (9521):** 1533–40.

7 Smith GS, Barss P. Unintentional injuries in developing countries: the epidemiology of a neglected problem. *Epidemiol Rev* 1991; **13:** 228–66.

8 Lane SD, Mikhail BI, Reizian A *et al.* Sociocultural aspects of blindness in an Egyptian delta hamlet: visual impairment vs. visual disability. *Med Anthropol* 1993; **15 (3):** 245–60.

9 Al-Lamki Z, Ohlin C. A community-based study of childhood handicap in Oman. *J Trop Pediatr* 1991; **38 (6):** 314–16.

10 Florian V, Shurka E. Jewish and Arab parents' coping patterns with their disabled child in Israel. *Int J Rehabil Res* 1981; **4 (2):** 201–4.

11 Shurka E, Florian V. A study of Israeli Jewish and Arab parental perceptions of their disabled children. *Journal of Comparative Family Studies* 1983; **14 (3):** 367–75.

12 Young Y. Families and the handicapped in northern Jordan. *Journal of Comparative Family Studies* 1997; **28 (2):** 151–69.

13 Shaar KH, McCarthy M. Disadvantage as a measure of handicap: a paired sibling study of disabled adults in Lebanon. *Int J Epidemiol* 1992; **21 (1):** 101–7.

14 Shurka E. Evaluation of persons with a physical disability: the influence of variables related to the disabled on Arab and Jewish youth. *Journal of Cross-Cultural Psychology* 1982; **13 (1):** 105–16.

15 Rosenbaum P, Stewart D. The World Health Organization International Classification of Functioning, Disability, and Health: a model to guide clinical thinking, practice and research in the field of cerebral palsy. *Semin Pediatr Neurol* 2004; **11 (1):** 5–10.

16 Rolland JS, Walsh F. Facilitating family resilience with childhood illness and disability. *Curr Opin Pediatr* 2006; **18 (5):** 527–38.

17 Reiter S, Mar'i S, Rosenberg Y. Parental attitudes toward the developmentally disabled among Arab communities in Israel: a cross-cultural study. *Int J Rehabil Res* 1986; **9 (4):** 355–62.

18 Milaat WA, Ghabrah TM, Al-Bar HM *et al.* Population-based survey of childhood disability in eastern Jeddah using the ten questions tool. *Disabil Rehabil* 2001; **23 (5):** 199–203.

19 Shawki S, Abalkhail B, Soliman N. An epidemiological study of childhood disability in Jeddah, Saudi Arabia. *Paediatric and Perinatal Epidemiology* 2002; **16 (1):** 61–6.

20 Eapen V, Zoubeidi T, Yunis F *et al.* Prevalence and psychosocial correlates of global developmental delay in 3-year-old children in the United Arab Emirates. *J Psychosom Res* 2006; **61 (3):** 321–6.

21 Duvdevany I, Abboud S. Stress, social support and well-being of Arab mothers of children with intellectual disability who are served by welfare services in northern Israel. *J Intellect Disabil Res* 2003; **47 (Pt 4–5):** 264–72.

22 Crabtree S. Maternal perceptions of care-giving of children with developmental disabilities in the United Arab Emirates. *Journal of Applied Research in Intellectual Disabilities* 2007; **20 (3):** 247–55.

23 Kandel I, Morad M, Vardi G *et al.* The Arab community in Israel coping with intellectual developmental disability. *The Scientific World Journal* 2004; **4:** 324–32.

24 Khamis V. Psychological distress among parents of children with mental retardation in the United Arab Emirates. *Soc Sci Med* 2007; **64 (4):** 850–7.

25 United Nations. *Proceedings of ESCWA Regional Seminar on the Role of the Family in Integrating Disabled Women into Society.* Amman; October 1994.

26 Alghazo E, Dodeen H, Algaryouti I. Attitudes of pre-service teachers towards persons with disabilities: predicting for the success of inclusion. *College Student Journal* 2003; **37 (4):** 515–22.

27 Alghazo E, El-Naggar Gaad E. General education teachers in the United Arab Emirates and their acceptance of the inclusion of students with disabilities. *British Journal of Special Education* 2004; **31 (2):** 94–9.

28 Lakkis S. Mobilising women with physical disabilities: the Lebanese Sitting Handicapped Association. In: Abu-Habib L, editor. *Gender and Disability: women's experiences in the Middle East.* Oxford: Oxfam; 1997.

CHAPTER 9

Age and aging

(★ *Abdelrazzak Abyad*

Introduction

The population of the world is aging. Many factors have resulted in increases in the numbers of elderly persons, including improvements in living standards, the curbing of communicable disease, and the latest breakthroughs in medical science.

It is currently estimated that more than half (58%) of all people who are 65 years and older live in developing nations. The world's older population experiences a net increase of 1.2 million each month, and 80% of this increase occurs in developing nations.[1-3] It is projected that by the year 2025, the total elderly population will reach 976 million and 72% of the elderly will live in developing regions.[2-4] Also, as is the case in developed countries, the growth rate is fastest for the oldest old, those most likely to have chronic diseases and be in need of health services. The Arab world will develop rapidly aging populations within the next few decades. Shrinking family sizes and social changes will reduce traditional family support for elders. The morbidity burden of the geriatric population can quickly overwhelm fragile and under-financed health infrastructures which are often unable to adequately meet prevention and treatment needs of a younger population with relatively low-cost, easy-to-prevent, easy-to-treat illnesses.

There is a critical need to define the policies and programs that will reduce the burden of aging populations on societies and economies. Therefore, the problems of the frail elderly, the development of geriatric programs and the education of professionals and para-professionals in geriatric principles are issues that will need to be addressed urgently.

Health transition

The Arab world is passing through a "health transition phase", characterized by an unprecedented increase in both number and proportion of adults and elderly persons. Improvement of healthcare has been achieved by a combination of technical advances, social organization, health expenditure and health education.[5-12] The epidemiological consequences of these changes will lead to increasing rates of death from cancer and circulatory disorders. In addition, an increase in chronic disorders of old age and increased medical needs of the aged will make enormous demands on the healthcare systems of the region. Geriatric care services for the elderly are generally unsatisfactory. Some countries in the region have started programs which, however, remain rudimentary and fragmented; no strong programs exist at a national level.[9-12]

Epidemiological data

There is a lack of appropriate knowledge about the nature and extent of health problems in the region. Statistics and data about health problems within the community are scarce. Much of our epidemiological knowledge of health problems comes from studies using hospitals or health services as data sources.

For these reasons, program priorities are often based on inappropriate or incomplete information.

Life expectancy

Life expectancy at birth reflects factors such as infant mortality, poor control of infectious diseases in childhood and youth, violent deaths, and genetic diseases leading to early mortality. Table 9.1 shows the life expectancy at birth for the region compared to other areas in the world. In the developed world, life expectancy is relatively increased for both genders (above 75 years for the United States and close to 80 years for Japan). The Arab countries show wide variations in their life expectancy, ranging from as high as 75 years in Kuwait to 63.9 years in Egypt and as low as 50.4 years in Yemen.[5-12]

However, when evaluating the health of elderly populations, estimations of life expectancy at age 65 years are a more accurate reflection of the adequacy of healthcare. Data reflecting life expectancy at age 65 are not readily available for Arab countries, but it is projected that the percentages of individuals classified as "elderly" in the Arab countries will grow substantially by 2050 (*see* Table 9.2).

Another important factor that is expected to compound demographic aging in many Arab countries is the ongoing emigration of young adults to developing countries for employment.[13] This will result in a higher dependency burden, where a growing percentage of elderly will be supported by diminishing numbers of economically active individuals.

TABLE 9.1 Life expectancy at birth for selected countries

LIFE EXPECTANCY AT BIRTH (YEARS)	MALES	FEMALES	TOTAL
Lebanon	66.8	70.7	68.7
Developed countries			
Japan	76.5	82.6	79.6
United States	72.6	79.4	76.1
Arab countries			
Kuwait	73.4	77.3	75.0
Saudi Arabia	68.6	71.6	69.9
Tunisia	67.1	68.9	68.0
Iraq	64.6	67.6	66.1
Egypt	62.7	65.1	63.9
Yemen	50.1	50.6	50.4
Developing countries			
Kenya	54.1	57.1	55.5
Nigeria	49.0	52.2	50.6
Angola	45.2	48.4	46.8
World	61.4	64.6	63.0

Compiled from UNDP *Human Development Report,* 1996.

Psychiatric morbidity

Psychiatric morbidity in the Arab world is underestimated, and few epidemiological studies have been carried out. Screening of representative samples of primary healthcare patients in Saudi Arabia and the United Arab Emirates (UAE) demonstrated psychiatric morbidity of 26% and 27.6% respectively.[12,14] Other data from elderly Bahraini[15] and Iraqi[16] primary care patients also demonstrated that significant proportions suffered from psychiatric problems, primarily depression. Studies of community-dwelling elders in Saudi Arabia,[17] Jordan[18] and the UAE[19] also suggest a high prevalence of psychiatric morbidity among these populations. A study from Israel comparing rates of psychological morbidity among elderly Muslims, Christians, Druze and Jews reported that, although rates of emotional distress were high, there were no clear differences in rates of suspected psychopathology among the four groups.[20]

Unofficial data from different nursing home facilities in Lebanon revealed a 25–30% level of depression among residents and 10–15% of dementia. At Ain WaZein elderly care center, Lebanon, dementia affects approximately 20% of the residents and depression is present in 25%. Behavioral disturbances affect around 20–30% of residents in long-term stay facilities in Lebanon. A study of institutionalized elderly in the UAE reported that 89% suffered from dementia.[21]

TABLE 9.2 Population aged 60 years and older in selected Arab countries in 2000 and projected in 2050

COUNTRY	% OF POPULATION AGED 60+ IN 2000	PROJECTED % OF POPULATION AGED 60+ IN 2050
Algeria	6	22.2
Bahrain	4.7	24.9
Egypt	6.3	20.8
Iraq	4.6	15.1
Jordan	4.5	15.6
Kuwait	4.4	25.7
Lebanon	8.5	25.4
Libya	5.5	21.1
Morocco	6.4	20.6
Palestine	4.9	9.9
Oman	4.2	10.5
Qatar	3.1	20.7
Saudi Arabia	4.8	12.9
Sudan	5.5	14.4
Syria	4.7	18.0
Tunisia	8.4	24.6
UAE	5.1	26.7
Yemen	3.6	5.3

Compiled from DESA. *World Population Aging 1950–2050* (New York: United Nations; 2002).

Socioeconomic and political factors

The aging of the population has been called a "great triumph of civilization", but it also presents the challenge of ensuring that older people have access to the economic, social and health resources that they need – a situation generally similar in developing nations to that of developed nations.[10] Suffering of the elderly may be severe, mainly because of poverty. Only a minority of elderly in the region benefit from pension systems.[13]

The extended family

Currently, the pressing problems for many elderly in the region are economic difficulties and low access to health services. By and large, there are few housing problems, since the traditional family still provides protection for the old.

The urban poor often manage to maintain extended families intact, though frequently in undesirable circumstances in slum housing. At the other end of the social scale, upper-income persons can afford the large homes and household help that allow them to accommodate all members of the extended family.[22] It is the middle income family, living in a nuclear household, frequently with the wife in the labor force, which is most likely to institutionalize an older relative. As the family is generally more effective and efficient than public institutions in caring for their elderly members, planning and social policy should encourage continued strong intergenerational relationships. Financial, social and emotional assistance to family members who care for their elderly relatives should be provided from governmental and non-governmental agencies.

Erosion of traditional family systems has been reported in recent years, due to factors such as youth migration for employment and increasing individualism. One study from Israel suggests that traditional supportive family interactions remain relatively unchanged among rural-dwelling Palestinian families.[23] Abuse and neglect of the elderly has been reported to be on the rise in some areas, including Saudi Arabia[24] and Israel.[25] A study among elderly Arabs in Israel suggests that increasing urbanization and decreased social integration of the elderly makes them more prone to victimization, neglect and abuse.[26]

Some authorities from developing countries challenge the assumption that families can continue to be depended on to take care of old people.[5–12,27,28]

One study revealed that suicide rates are higher among elderly people living in three-generation households than among those living alone.[29]

Future research in the Arab world should explore the changing roles of the elderly within the family, and attitudes toward the old.

The status of the elderly in Arab culture

Middle-Eastern culture ensures respect for the elderly and values highly the natural bonds of affection between all members of the family. The eldest members are a source of spiritual blessing, religious faith, wisdom and love. Despite the general feeling among most people in the region that sending an elderly parent to a nursing home violates their sacred sense of duty toward them,[30] many families are faced with situations where they have no other alternative. It is clear that the majority of elderly persons in nursing and psychiatric homes are there owing to circumstances with which their families are unable to cope – including the families' living abroad, their inability to support their elders financially, and the nature of the diseases from which the elderly suffer and which require professional care. Although rates of institutionalization of older adults are lower in the Arab world than in Western nations, institutionalized adults tend to be far more dependent and in need of specialized care than do nursing home patients in developed countries.[21,31] This pattern will continue to worsen as morbidity patterns change, leading to longer life spans with chronic disease, dependency and loss of autonomy for growing numbers of elderly in the region.

Elderly people in the area receive much social and economic support from extended kin networks – particularly from their own children. With smaller families being the trend, fewer potentially supportive children will be available to care for the elderly. Studies from developed countries show that where children are in a position to help their aged parents, the majority of them do so. However, traditional patterns of family responsibility are likely to diminish with economic development.[29] Young city dwellers may become more preoccupied with the future of their children than with the difficulties of their parents. Women, who have customarily played major roles in providing family care, are increasingly entering the labor force out of personal choice and economic necessity, and may no longer be available to care for aged relatives.[5–12,27,28]

The political situation

Governments in the area continue to assume that families will continue to take care of their own elderly members, despite objective projections indicating that long-term care will be an important part of healthcare planning in the future.[2] Governments are often unwilling or unable to make major commitments to elderly health.[5–12,27–9]

In Egypt, for example, there are only 34 "old people's homes" for a population of over one million elderly people. Some homes are reported to have waiting lists of over 1000 persons.

Indeed, if present economic trends continue, governments may be even less able to adequately finance programs and healthcare for the elderly. This is particularly problematic, as medical interventions for older individuals, whether preventive or curative, are typically far more expensive than healthcare for younger populations.[5,10,27,32–4] Increasing conflicts will arise between the needs of large population groups and the purchasing power of a limited elite.

Given the fragile finances of many governments, the private sector may play a greater role in the future of elder care in the region. Already, most of the programs that exist in the region have been developed at the community level or by the private sector.

When considering options for the future, the countries in the Arab world can be divided into the following groups:

- countries typified by substantial capital, rapid development and a small indigenous population – such as Saudi Arabia, Kuwait and most of the Gulf states
- countries with less capital, more people, a quantitatively larger medical infrastructure, and more trained medical personnel – such as Egypt, Israel and Algeria
- countries whose extensive medical service plans have been halted or greatly decreased in scope because of civil strife or war – such as Iraq, Lebanon and Palestine.[11]

Each group of countries will need to assess its strengths and weaknesses to determine how best to meet the challenges of the demographic transition in their region. For some, emphasis on western-style institutions and structures may be optimal, for others, renewed efforts to retain traditional care patterns of the elderly will be required. In most, a combination of approaches, or novel approaches may be developed.

Characteristics of the elderly

"Diversity" is a key term that describes the elderly population. While the label "elderly" is commonly used for the population aged 65 years and over, this group is remarkably heterogeneous. Each age, gender and ethnic group has distinctive characteristics, and the experience of aging differs among demographic groups. For example, the rural elderly have characteristics and needs that differ from those of urban-dwelling elderly. Some older people have significant health problems while others spend time vacationing, exercising and participating in sports. Some stay in the paid workforce until they die, while others fill their leisure time with volunteer work, care for children and frailer elderly persons than themselves, or other personally satisfying activities. Some are bored, angry or depressed. In short, the elderly, like other age groups, include people with varied levels of needs, abilities and resources.

Clinical assessment of the elderly

As individuals grow older, the goals of health maintenance expand from a primary focus on preventing and treating disease to one that includes maximization of quality of life, preservation of productivity and independence, and attaining satisfaction with life. It is important for the clinician to actively seek out and periodically evaluate a number of medical and social areas. Older people are often slow to bring these to the clinician's attention, because the complaints are vague, or they accept disability as a part of old age. Early detection and treatment of abnormalities is important. For example, patients who are detected in the early stage of mobility difficulties may be sent for rehabilitation before they fall and suffer a fracture, or become deconditioned and bed-bound. Those who are found to suffer from dementia at early stages will benefit from advance planning for care with the family, and possibly medications to slow progression of the condition.

Areas that should be assessed regularly include:
- *mobility and activities of daily living:* among activities of daily living (ADLs) are the individual's basic abilities to: Dress themselves, Eat, Ambulate, Toilet and maintain Hygiene or bathe (DEATH). In addition, elders who live independently should be evaluated for instrumental activities of daily living (IADLs), which include: Shopping, Housekeeping, Accounting (or the ability to handle and keep track of finances), Food preparation and Transportation (SHAFT)
- *medications:* about 15% of hospitalizations of elderly individuals in Western countries are due to adverse drug reactions. As individuals age, they become

more sensitive to the effects of many medications, and are unable to metabolize them as efficiently as younger people. In addition, older individuals often require many different types of medications for different ailments. This increases the risk of drug–drug interactions

➴ *mentation:* the prevalence of dementia in the Arab world is poorly studied. Dementia prevalence has been reported to be as high as 20.5% among some elderly Palestinian populations[35] and as low as 1.4% in Assiut, Egypt.[36] Early detection of dementia is important. People with dementia often develop it insidiously over several years, and are prone to the consequences of poor judgment and injuries arising as a result

➴ *hearing and vision:* both hearing and vision decline with age in all individuals. Early detection and correction of low vision or hearing can improve patient safety and quality of life

➴ *incontinence:* incontinence in the elderly, both to urine and stool, is a frequent problem. Urinary incontinence has been reported to be particularly common among elderly women; however, very few report this to the physician because of embarrassment[37]

➴ *nutrition:* problems with nutrition among the elderly are common. Factors as varied as poor dentition, poverty and malabsorption can all lead to malnutrition

➴ *depression:* as outlined above, elderly patients frequently suffer from psychiatric distress and depression. A low threshold of suspicion for this condition is important in the clinical setting. Patients with chronic medical conditions – such as chronic obstructive lung disease, diabetes or post-stroke – are at particular risk of developing depression.

Facilities for the elderly

It is well accepted that social, environmental and psychological factors can influence ill-health among the elderly as much as can biological factors. Bereavement, social isolation, loss of work roles, lack of physical activity, poor nutrition and misuse of medicines constitute major risk factors for illness and premature death. Therefore the priority is the provision of medical, psychiatric and rehabilitative services for early diagnosis and treatment of these conditions in order to reduce morbidity. It is important to achieve a balance of care between community and institutional services, both for humanitarian and economic reasons. Given the demographic factors mentioned above, the need for long-term care services will undoubtedly grow, including nursing facilities as well as home or community-based long-term care. Accurate information about the conditions and needs of older persons is crucial for planning health service development and training of personnel. Of primary importance is determination of the age distribution of older populations, since there are marked differences between the health and resource needs of groups in the "young aged" category and the more vulnerable "extreme aged" (80 and over).

An interesting observation from research in the region is the contribution of social visitation and integration to the well-being of Arab elders. Studies suggest that ongoing social interaction and belonging to a strong social network is a major factor resulting in successful aging among elders in the region, and may be perceived to be even more important than optimal physical functioning.[38–41] There has been a reported resurgence of community-based clubs where older individuals go to socialize.[42] This is an example of an ongoing cultural tradition that may be encouraged to improve health and well-being of older individuals at low cost.

Education and training
Role of academic institutions

One of the most important areas in caring for the elderly is to focus on the need for geriatric and gerontological education and training for a wide range of health professionals and para-professionals who provide care to elderly persons, in order to meet the future demand for quality, long-term care services.

Currently, there is a limited supply of well-trained primary care physicians and major deficiencies in local training in geriatrics, occupational or environmental health, and preventive medicine.[5,9–11]

Medical schools in the area generally press for strong basic science programs and sophisticated tertiary care, and there is a trend toward sub-specialization. There is a need for schools to modify their curricula to address national or local health needs, to emphasize primary healthcare and preventive medicine, and to prepare health professionals to be responsive to demographic changes. Few academic institutions seem focused on the demographic, social or medical problems associated with an aging population. Many are in a mid-twentieth-century mode, patterned after traditional schools in the developed world, and there is little emphasis on curricular content or research involving the aged and aging. The recent development of a Family Medicine Program with community orientation appropriate to the resources – cultural, material and economic – available in the community, however, is encouraging.[5,9–11]

Geriatrics vs gerontology

There is substantial overlap between "geriatrics" and "gerontology", but these terms are not synonymous. Geriatrics refers to the clinical practice by physicians and other healthcare professionals involved in treating elderly patients. On the other hand, gerontology is the inter-disciplinary study of older persons, including fields such as economics, psychology, sociology, political science and many other academic and applied areas. It is critical that healthcare providers, both professionals and para-professionals, understand both geriatric care and gerontology. That is, in addition to knowing about the diseases and conditions being treated, they also need to know about older individuals, both as people and as patients. They need to know how to effectively communicate with older persons, how to be supportive and to appropriately respond to their complex array of concerns and problems.

The increasing need for geriatric education and training in the region will be driven by changing demographics. A rising geriatric population, with increasingly unmet healthcare needs, strongly advocates for better educational preparation of those health professionals serving them. The absence of sufficient numbers of trained geriatricians and gerontologists, among other health professionals, seriously undermines the ability of a country's healthcare system to adequately assess, treat and rehabilitate the aged. This shortage will lead to inappropriate care, higher costs and poorer patient outcomes. Education is key in optimizing available resources.

Health professionals

Few health professionals have received training in the care of the elderly, and many do not find working with them to be rewarding. This often leads to avoidance of older people and their problems. Clinical training of health professionals should include participation in interdisciplinary work in order to gain knowledge and appreciation of the roles of all health and social service workers, to be better able to work as a team. The needs of older adults, especially the frail or impaired, require a healthcare workforce knowledgeable about the systems and services of care with which the elderly interact, and the skills to provide care within these systems. Care of the elderly, within managed care and long-term care systems, requires a unique body of knowledge and experience to be able to work cooperatively with managers and other members of the care team. Systems should develop rewards, both professional and financial, for those who work with the elderly.

The complexity of problems common to older adults often demands knowledge and skills beyond those possessed by individual practitioners; involving a range of health professionals and para-professionals in providing care to elderly persons will contribute to the provision of high-quality services.[5,9–11]

These changes will have far-reaching effects in the near future, when it is anticipated that much of a healthcare professional's time will be devoted to care for the elderly. A health workforce, prepared with the knowledge base and technical skills of geriatrics and gerontology, can respond more effectively and efficiently to the needs that arise with advancing age. There is no doubt that, through research, education and training, a skilled workforce can help reduce disability and functional limitations, improve the quality of life for both the aged and their family members, and can be an effective means of providing appropriate healthcare to an aging society.

Implications for nursing

As this century progresses, nurses in the Arab world will be increasingly concerned with the aging population. Nursing must focus upon the entire spectrum of health and develop interventions geared not only toward the individual patient, but also toward the family and community. The nursing profession is ideally placed to encourage elderly people to optimize their physical, social and psychological function during changes in their state of health.

The key allowing the nursing profession to effectively cope with the challenges of caring for the elderly lies in specialized training that equips nurses with the knowledge needed for this task. There are no gerontological nurses in the region. There is a need for nurses to stress emphasis on health rather than illness,[43] in addition to stressing the holistic aspect of nursing practice with older adults.[44] There is also a need to incorporate gerontological nursing preparation into basic nursing education.[45] The development of a Nursing Home Program is of vital importance. It will help nursing homes gain access to the research and educational resources of universities, with student access to actual clinical nursing situations in real-world settings.

Nurses who care for geriatric patients are primary care and frontline providers. They coordinate and manage the care of the aged. The role of the geriatric nurse, in primary and managed care settings, can best be described as that of the healthcare provider who assesses the clients' needs and strengths on an ongoing basis, and provides continuity and coordination of care and referrals to appropriate health professionals and agencies. Nursing in this context is largely focused on health promotion, disease prevention and long-term management of chronic disorders and their exacerbations which often require triage for prompt and intensive interventions.

Social work

Similar to the above-mentioned professions, the need for social services for the elderly will be increasing in the next few decades. A recent survey from the United States concluded that geriatric social work is among the fastest growing specializations within the profession. Similarly, in the Arab world there will be increasing needs for social, emotional and environmental support services for the elderly. Concomitantly, there will be an even greater need for geriatric social work education. Social workers are key members of the interdisciplinary team required to deal with the complex problems of older persons. This teamwork recognizes that such problems necessitate a comprehensive and planned approach to their resolution.

Geriatric social work is built on a bio-psychosocial theoretical foundation. This includes an emphasis on the person in a sociocultural context, where an individual is conceptualized as a member of a kinship group, a family system and an informal system including neighbors and friends. Coping with illness and disability is viewed within the context of this system primarily, but includes the formal service delivery system and its interface with the informal system. The inter-relationship of social, psychological, biological and economic factors in determining the situations of older people, and the nature of their needs, makes a team approach to professional practice and service delivery essential. From the beginnings of the profession, social workers have always taken responsibility for what is now called *case management*; that is, the responsibility to help secure the resources that older adults need in a timely and appropriate fashion. Similarly, they have taken responsibility for facilitating the linkages among agencies and inaugurating a system in order to ensure continuity of services. Among the benefits to the elderly person are coordinated services, the ability to access more skilled services, avoidance of duplication of services, and convenience.

Today, case management is an essential component of the provision of care to older people, partly because of the fragmentation and discontinuities in the service delivery system, and partly because of the emphasis on cost efficiency and effectiveness. Although other professions are engaged in the provision of case management, the expertise of geriatric social workers continues to be a strong justification for the centrality of their role as case managers, and for their inclusion on geriatric interdisciplinary teams.

Education on the role of case management, which is designed to contain healthcare costs and improve the quality of care delivered, should be emphasized. Also, increasing emphasis should be placed on community-based geriatric services, on preparing geriatric social workers for work with families and communities to facilitate linkage with the formal health system, and on advocacy as well as other roles.

Solutions and future directions

Two expert committees from the World Health Organization (WHO)[46,47] have suggested that the sophisticated and specialized services for the elderly found in the developed world are irrelevant for the immediate future and may not even be appropriate as long-term objectives in developing countries. Consequently, the WHO has developed a tentative model to meet the needs of the elderly citizens in developing nations.[48] In this model, the needs of elderly people are, as far as possible, met within the system of care developed for the population as a whole. Patterns of care are based on functional assessment of the elderly. This model envisages a system of care built up from the primary care resources of the community. Special emphasis is given to programs that assist the family in its traditional role of supporting the elderly. Institutional long-term care services are made available only when other alternatives are exhausted.

The severely impaired and dependent aged will need a wide range of professional care, as will their families. In the process of creating adequate services, it is important to realize that home care and institutional services are complementary and multidirectional. Care of such patients needs the shared responsibility of both families and professional service providers. Services can be provided in the home, the community, the institution or any combination of these settings.

The role of those concerned with aging in the Arab world is to provide communities and concerned professionals with the knowledge and skills to solve their problems, and not to import solutions from developed countries before other alternatives have been explored. Health promotion and prevention should be key factors in any program. Geriatric and gerontological information should be a part of the education of all health professionals. Environmental design of hospitals and clinics should take into consideration the needs of the elderly.

Public awareness

Aging is a biological process. It is not a disease. In order to increase the population's awareness of it, it is important to provide accurate information on the needs and abilities of older people. Bringing gerontological content to the school curriculum of children as preparation for adult life is one alternative to improve the public image of elderly patients. Many youngsters show signs of prejudice against older persons – an attitude that is now called "ageism".[49]

Research

Despite the fact that 93% of potential years of life lost are in developing countries, only 5% of all research funds are spent on the health problems of these countries.[2] Research is needed to optimize the potential of older persons and to improve their opportunities to perform rewarding roles in society.

Conclusion

The demographic, medical and social changes with subsequent unprecedented growth of the elderly population are creating new realities in the Arab world. Such trends as rapid urbanization, movement away from traditional family structures and ongoing technological development make the problem of aging in the Middle East an acute one. Widespread and inappropriate applications of costly technologies will result in diversion of scarce resources from existing primary care services to the overall detriment of the existing healthcare system. Changes in national policies and priorities, educational curricula and research, will all be critical steps to ensure the best possible quality of life for the greatest possible number of our aged.

References

1 Anon. *World Population Prospects: estimates and projections as assessed in 1982.* New York: United Nations; 1985. pp. 4–14.

2 Kinsella K. *Aging in the Third World.* Center for International Research; 1988.

3 World Health Organization. *World Health Statistics Annual.* Geneva: World Health Organization; 1996. pp. 171–7.

4 *Health of the Elderly.* Geneva: World Health Organization; 1997.

5 Abyad A. Geriatrics in Lebanon: the beginning. *Int J Aging Hum Dev* 1995; **41 (4):** 299–309.

6 Courbage Y, Fargues P. La situation démographique au Liban. In: *Mortalité, fécondité et projections; méthodes et résultats.* Beyrouth: Imprimerie Catholique; 1973. p. 104.

7 Faour N. The demography of Lebanon: a reappraisal. *Journal of Middle Eastern Studies* 1991; **27 (4):** 631–41.

8 Kronfol N, Mroueh A. *Health Care in Lebanon.* Alexandria: WHO; 1984.

9 Abyad A. The Lebanese health care system. *Fam Pract* 1994; **11 (2):** 159–61.

10 Abyad A. Geriatrics in the Middle East: the challenges. *The Practitioner* (Eastern Mediterranean edition) 1995; **6 (12):** 869–70.

11 Abyad A. Family medicine in the Middle East: reflections on the experiences of several countries. *J Am Board Fam Pract* 1996; **9 (4):** 289–97.

12 Abyad A. Health care for older persons: a country profile – Lebanon. *J Am Geriatr Soc* 2001; **49 (10):** 1366–70.

13 *Ageing in the Arab Countries: regional variations, policies and programmes.* 2004 [cited 2007, 21 February]. Available from: www.escwa.org.lb/information/publications/sdd/docs/04-wg-1-2.pdf

14 El-Rufaie OE, Absood GH. Minor psychiatric morbidity in primary health care: prevalence, nature and severity. *Int J Soc Psychiatry* 1993; **39 (3):** 159–66.

15 Al Haddad M. Depression in primary care attendees in Bahrain. *Arab Journal of Psychiatry* 2000; **11 (1):** 48–55.

16 Ali N, Hussien A. Depression in elderly patients attending primary health care clinics in Baghdad City. *Arab Journal of Psychiatry* 2005; **16 (2):** 107–17.

17 Abolfotouh MA, Daffallah AA, Khan MY *et al.* Psychosocial assessment of geriatric subjects in Abha City, Saudi Arabia. *East Mediterr Health J* 2001; **7 (3):** 481–91.

18 Youssef RM. Comprehensive health assessment of senior citizens in Al-Karak governorate, Jordan. *East Mediterr Health J* 2005; **11 (3):** 334–48.

19 Ghubash R, El-Rufaie O, Zoubeidi T *et al.* Profile of mental disorders among the elderly United Arab Emirates population: sociodemographic correlates. *Int J Geriatr Psychiatry* 2004; **19 (4):** 344–51.

20 Shemesh AA, Kohn R, Blumstein T *et al.* A community study on emotional distress among Arab and Jewish Israelis over the age of 60. *Int J Geriatr Psychiatry* 2006; **21 (1):** 64–76.

21 Margolis SA, Reed RL. Institutionalized older adults in a health district in the United Arab Emirates: health status and utilization rate. *Gerontology* 2001; **47 (3):** 161–7.

22 Margolis SA, Carter T, Dunn EV *et al.* The health status of community based elderly in the United Arab Emirates. *Arch Gerontol Geriatr* 2003; **37 (1):** 1–12.

23 Weihl H. Household, family and intergenerational interaction of rural Arab elderly in Israel. *Journal of Cross-Cultural Gerontology* 2004; **3 (2):** 121–38.

24 Ashy M. Saudi Arabia. In: Malley-Morrison K, editor. *International Perspectives on Family Violence and Abuse: a cognitive ecological approach.* Mahwah, New Jersey: Lawrence Erlbaum Associates, Publishers; 2004. p. 180.

25 Siegel-Itzkovich J. A fifth of elderly people in Israel are abused. *BMJ* 2005; **330 (7490):** 498.

26 Litwin H, Zoabi S. Modernization and elder abuse in an Arab-Israeli context. *Research on Aging* 2003; **25 (3):** 224–46.

27 *Population and Development: the demographic profile of Arab countries.* New York: United Nations; 2003.

28 Courbage Y, Fargues P. Some methodological elements proper to Lebanese data (1970) in order to obtain indices on mortality. In: Expert Group Meeting on Mortality. Beirut, Lebanon: UNESOB and WHO; 1972. p. 21.

29 *World Population Projects.* New York: United Nations; 1991.

30 Fitzgerald M, Mullavey-O'Bryne C, Clemson L. Families and nursing home placements: a cross-cultural study. *Journal of Cross-Cultural Geriatrics* 2001; **16:** 333–51.

31 Suleiman K, Walter-Ginzburg A. A nursing home in Arab-Israeli society: targeting utilization in a changing social and economic environment. *J Am Geriatr Soc* 2005; **53 (1):** 152–7.

32 Armenian HK, Halabi SS, Khlat M. Epidemiology of primary health problems in Beirut. *J Epidemiol Community Health* 1989; **43 (4):** 315–18.

33 Abyad A, Zoorob R, Sidani S. "Family Medicine" in Lebanon: the 10th anniversary. *Fam Med* 1992; **24 (8):** 575–9.

34 Kronfol N, Mroueh A. *Health Care in Lebanon.* Beirut: Makassed Press; 1985. pp. 440–50.

35 Bowirrat A, Treves TA, Friedland RP *et al.* Prevalence of Alzheimer's type dementia in an elderly Arab population. *Eur J Neurol* 2001; **8 (2):** 119–23.

36 Farrag A, Farwiz HM, Khedr EH *et al.* Prevalence of Alzheimer's disease and other dementing disorders: Assiut-Upper Egypt study. *Dement Geriatr Cogn Disord* 1998; **9 (6):** 323–8.

37 Rizk DE, Shaheen H, Thomas L *et al.* The prevalence and determinants of health care-seeking behavior for urinary incontinence in United Arab Emirates women. *Int Urogynecol J Pelvic Floor Dysfunct* 1999; **10 (3):** 160–5.

38 Litwin H. Correlates of successful aging: are they universal? *Int J Aging Hum Dev* 2005; **61 (4):** 313–33.

39 Litwin H. The path to well-being among elderly Arab Israelis. *J Cross-Cult Gerontol* 2006; **21 (1–2):** 25–40.

40 Litwin H. Social networks and self-rated health: a cross-cultural examination among older Israelis. *J Aging Health* 2006; **18 (3):** 335–58.

41 Sabbah I, Drouby N, Sabbah S *et al.* Quality of life in rural and urban populations in Lebanon using SF-36 health survey. *Health Qual Life Outcomes* 2003; **1 (1):** 30.

42 Azaiza F, Brodsky J. The aging of Israel's Arab population: needs, existing responses, and dilemmas in the development of services for a society in transition. *Isr Med Assoc J* 2003; **5 (5):** 383–6.

43 Surveillance and Monitoring Project, WHO. *Weekly Epidemiological Record* 1984; **59:** 122–3.

44 Emergency Health Surveillance Project, July–November 1982, WHO. *Weekly Epidemiological Record* 1986; **58:** 7–9.

45 Lockwood L, Armenian HK, Zurayk H. A population based survey of loss and psychological distress during war. *Soc Sci Med* 1986; **23:** 269–75.

46 Nuwayhid I, Sibai A, Adib S *et al.* Morbidity, mortality and risk factors. In: Deeb M, editor. *Beirut: a health profile.* Beirut: American University of Beirut; 1997. pp. 30–45.

47 Kronfol N, Mroueh A. *Health Care in Lebanon.* Beirut: WHO; 1985. pp. 440–50.
48 Martin LG. The aging of Asia. *J Gerontol* 1988; **43 (4):** S99–113.
49 Evand J. The discovery of the aged in the Third World. *Acad Med* 1989; **64:** 76–8.

CHAPTER 10

Death and dying

(★ Laeth S Nasir

Introduction

It is generally recognized that dealing with medical issues surrounding death and dying is among the most challenging tasks for physicians in any part of the world. Until recently, very little literature or research was available to help guide physicians and others in managing and understanding end-of-life issues.

Some issues that surround death are very individual and culture-specific; particularly in Arab countries, the diversity of religions, traditions, culture change and the lack of research in this area all contribute to the complexity of the challenges faced by the clinician. It is important that this issue be thoroughly studied in the Arab world since death is unavoidable; understanding the social and cultural issues surrounding it, and successful management of this process by the physician, will go a long way to ameliorate suffering in the patient and his or her family.

The knowledge or threat of impending death can be one of the most stressful events in human experience. The emotional intensity and anxiety that this situation elicits can result in misconceptions, misjudgments and anger that may be directed at the physician. Given the large potential number of individual and unique combinations of fears, concerns and coping skills that patients and families may have, it can be difficult to predict what kind of reaction can be expected in response to death and dying.

Part of the physician's responsibility in dealing with death and dying is delivering bad news to patients and families. This task can be a difficult one for the physician; causing discomfort runs contrary to the provision of healing, comfort and protection that are traditionally seen as components of the physician's role. Very frequently in Arab countries, the physician will face families who will request that the physician not inform the patient of a grave diagnosis. Often, the family perceives that delivering a "death sentence" to the patient may actually harm his or her chances for survival and will to live.

This chapter will attempt to explore some of the medical issues involved in death and dying in Arab countries, and suggest directions for future practice and research.

Traditional and changing responses

Social responses to death in traditional Arab society are well developed and generally effective in mobilizing social and material support for the bereaved. Imminent or actual death triggers a familiar and organized series of rituals and responses from friends and family. These traditions are helpful in facilitating the normal grieving process.[1,2] The ability of physicians to accurately predict adverse outcomes at ever earlier stages of disease, and the capacity to sustain a moribund patient on life-support for long periods, have produced new states and subsequently new social realities. Examples of these states include the patient who is apparently perfectly well or only somewhat ill, yet has a substantial chance of dying, or the patient who is on life-support and stands little or no chance of survival, for whom a decision to possibly withdraw life-support needs to be made. For these scenarios, society does not yet have a well-developed "script" that provides tangible direction and social support. At times in fact, patients who are known to be suffering from a fatal illness such as cancer may experience a loss of social support due to the stigma and fear surrounding the diagnosis.[3]

Historically, the social stigma arising from fatal diagnoses was felt to be so strong that, in some countries, death certificates were designed so that the cause of death was written on a separate paper from the certificate itself. In this way, the family of the deceased would not feel stigmatized.[4,5]

Communication of a grave prognosis by physicians

Culture has a great influence on how or whether a grave prognosis is discussed with patients and their families. In many Western industrialized countries, patient autonomy is emphasized, with the expectation of full disclosure and discussion of the prognosis with the patient. Disclosure in this cultural context is essential in order to obtain consent for treatment, and to allow the patient control in making choices regarding his or her care. Practices around disclosure of disease differ in many other countries of the world, however, where a more nuanced and family-centered approach is often followed. In Japan, for example, physicians are far less likely than physicians in the United States to agree that a patient should be told about an incurable cancer diagnosis before telling his or her family.[6,7] For this reason, the late emperor of Japan was not told that he suffered from pancreatic cancer prior to his death.[8] A study that compared responses of 40 internists practicing in the United States and China found that 95% of the US physicians and none of the Chinese physicians would disclose a terminal cancer diagnosis to a hypothetical patient in a clinical vignette.[9] Studies from many other countries – including Italy, Greece, Spain, as well as several in South America and Africa – report similar findings.[10,11]

Communication of a grave prognosis in Arab countries

A number of studies have been carried out in Arab countries that explore the disclosure preferences and practices of physicians when faced by a patient with a grave prognosis. A study from Lebanon reported that only 47% of physicians surveyed would "usually" disclose a cancer diagnosis directly to a patient. Fewer than 20% of physicians in this study reported that their training or medical education had been a factor influencing their disclosure policy, although many had received their medical training in countries where disclosure was the norm. Rather, they reported that they had settled on their policy based on their own clinical experience and personal values. Most of the physicians said that they made occasional exceptions to their usual disclosure practice.[12] Another study from Kuwait reported that 79% of physicians felt that the diagnosis should be withheld if it was requested by the family. Interestingly, a personal experience of cancer involving a family member or friend increased the likelihood that the physician would be in favor of withholding the diagnosis.[13] In Saudi Arabia, only 47% of physicians surveyed would consistently provide diagnostic or prognostic information to a patient with a grave prognosis. Two-thirds preferred to disclose only to family. Physicians who were of more senior status were more likely to favor disclosure.[14] In the United Arab Emirates (UAE), a study comparing responses of patients and physicians found that although patients were statistically more likely than physicians to favor disclosure of a terminal prognosis when faced with a hypothetical scenario, the differences were not great.[15] A survey of 498 individuals that included 88 cancer outpatients, 99 non-cancer outpatients and 300 "healthy" individuals who were visiting healthcare facilities in Lebanon found that 42% generally preferred that the truth not be told to patients having a serious diagnosis. Younger individuals, individuals with more education and cancer patients were more likely to favor disclosure.[16] Younger people, and those with a family history of cancer, were also more likely to favor disclosure in a study from Saudi Arabia.[17] Arabs living in the United States tended, too, to hold the view that patients should not be told "bad news" regarding their illness.[18]

Taken together, these findings suggest that while physicians often do not disclose a terminal prognosis directly to patients, they may be responding at least in part to cultural expectations held by patients and their families. Some of the studies suggest a cohort effect, with younger individuals being more likely to express positive attitudes towards disclosure.

Ways of communicating bad news

For the physician, communicating bad news is never easy, even after years of practice. It is often helpful to plan the encounter beforehand, but this cannot always be assured, especially in the case of sudden unexpected death. The usual practice of communicating news of a grave diagnosis in Western countries is to provide direct information clearly and calmly. The use of the simplest language possible is important to maximize understanding. My usual practice is to try to communicate the diagnosis and prognosis several times during the meeting, since anxiety and denial are often present, and misunderstandings are very frequent. Calm avoidance of arguments about the diagnosis and side-issues is important; in the initial meeting only a limited number of topics should be addressed to avoid information "overload". It is important to acknowledge that it is difficult to predict how long an individual patient will survive. However, you can provide statements such as: "Most people with this condition will survive between three and six months." It is important to expect and to calmly allow people to express their expressions of grief and upset.

Regular meetings should be set up in order to answer questions, and to manage emotional issues and concerns.

Alternative methods of communicating a grave diagnosis exist, although these are not as well documented in the literature. Sometimes, when faced with a situation in which the physician is unsure whether or not the patient wants disclosure of the illness, it may be helpful to ask the patient directly how and to whom the information should be disclosed. For example: "Would you like me to tell you the full details of your condition – or is there someone else you would like me to talk to?" or "Do you like to know exactly what is going on, or would you prefer me to give you the outline only?"[19] Though this technique appears to be awkward and transparent, it is often very effective and usually meets the patient and family needs for "non-disclosure", while providing indirect notice of a serious condition.

Another method that has been described is an approach in which the physician communicates the diagnosis indirectly to the patient and family. To an outsider, this process appears to be primarily emotion-focused rather than information-focused. Although this approach requires in-depth cultural knowledge and linguistic skill to perform competently, it may be effective in providing patients with the level of knowledge that they require in order to make decisions about their own illness or in providing family with similar information about the illness of their loved one.[20,21] There is an urgent need for more research into these issues in Arab countries.

Patient and family responses to grave illness

Perceptions of illness and responses to illness are in large part socially determined. To understand the dynamics surrounding the range of individual and family responses to death and dying, it may be useful to explore different cultural narratives (shared perceptions, stories, symbolism and beliefs) that govern society's views of the meaning of life, illness and death.

Two prominent contrasting narratives that have been advanced are the "autonomy-control narrative" and the "social-embeddedness narrative". These patterns have been proposed by anthropologists to explain differences in living patterns and traditions in different parts of the world. While these worldviews may have been quite distinct in different cultures in the past, in our increasingly globalized world, the dichotomous adoption of one or the other narrative may not be the norm. Instead, attitudes and beliefs may vary with bits and parts of different cultural traditions existing simultaneously within the same family or individual.[22]

The "autonomy-control" narrative is currently the dominant one in many Western industrialized nations. In this model, society is seen as a collection of individuals, each of whom has his or her own separate and defined rights and interests. It is assumed that the individual alone knows what is right for him or her, and is expected to take full responsibility for the decisions that he or she makes. In addition, this worldview affirms that life and its problems are largely predictable and controllable; all problems are able to be solved through sufficient applications of logic, science, technology and the "right attitude". One's life, future and even death are seen as things to be evaluated, planned and manipulated. In the case of a serious illness, it is only necessary for the patient to understand the problem clearly, make a decision, marshal his or her resources and take action. Therefore, the role of the physician is to provide the most accurate information and allow the patient to choose. Communication is seen primarily as a means for information transfer; therefore, factual "objective" and concise forms of communication are emphasized. Withholding information or choices is seen as a violation of human rights, paternalistic, and an interference in the patient's control of their life.[23]

In contrast, individuals living in the setting of a "social-embeddedness" narrative perceive themselves as relational beings, rooted in a family and group that provides support, protection and a sense of meaning and continuity. Relationships are the fundamental reality of life, and the yardstick against which everything else is measured. Hierarchy is a given, beginning with the relationship between God and man, and extending to all other relationships. Interests and goals of the individual and group are not perceived to be divergent, so maintaining social unity is a fundamental value.[23] In order to strengthen and defend this unity, there is an emphasis on such behaviors as loyalty, duty and respect for authority. Maintenance of social harmony and propriety extends to communication style, which tends to be emotion-focused, indirect and subtle, with a tendency to overlook or conceal the unpleasant or uncomfortable aspects of a situation.

Rather than believing that life can be infinitely manipulated, this narrative emphasizes the fragility and unpredictable nature of existence and the importance of fate and God's will. Since life is ultimately mysterious and not controllable, having a choice and control over one's destiny are not fundamentally important. Although suffering cannot be avoided, it can be reduced and given meaning through the intervention and support of the family. Life is to be lived, not planned or controlled; adapting oneself to the vicissitudes of life with honor and grace is highly valued. Worrying about what will happen in the future is not valuable or rational.[23]

In this setting, non-disclosure can be seen as reverting to a more familiar and comforting style of coping – maintaining social cohesion through drawing the patient closer into the protective embrace of family to counter the "external" threat. An individual with a serious illness needs hope, comfort and the attentions of family to distract and comfort him or her. Disclosure of a serious illness to the affected individual in these circumstances seems dangerous and cruel.[23]

Very often, in spite of family efforts, the patient is able to guess or infer the diagnosis or prognosis without explicitly being told, and a pattern develops in which each party "protects" the other. One shields the patient against explicitly disclosing a diagnosis that is felt to take away all hope and the will to live, and the other shields the family from the anguish of knowing that he or she knows the diagnosis. For many families, this pattern may be adaptive; the emotionally soothing effect of social closeness and familiarity with the roles played outweighs the disadvantages of explicit disclosure. On the other hand, the parties may become increasingly isolated from one another, and the needs of both to plan and express wants and needs may be affected. In caring for these patients, providers should be alert to this type of dysfunction by monitoring dynamics and anxiety within the family and providing support as needed.

Patient and family responses to grave illness in Arab countries

A few studies have explored the attitudes and responses of Arab patients and their families in response to grave illness, most commonly cancer. A diagnosis of cancer is one of the most emotionally charged diagnoses in any culture – often symbolizing hopelessness, pain, suffering and death. Even in parts of the world where the most advanced treatments are available and patients have high levels of health literacy, cancer is a uniquely feared diagnosis.

The highly stigmatized status of cancer in Arab countries was demonstrated by a study of cancer patients in Egypt, in which the authors reported that they were unable to use the word "cancer" in questioning patients about their condition for fear of causing offense.[24]

Arab families' willingness to mobilize remarkable levels of support for patients with cancer or other serious illness is well documented in the literature.[25-7] This support can be so unqualified and overwhelming that it elicits guilt feelings in the patient. In a study that compared the attitudes and needs of cancer patients in the United States and Egypt, one of the top three needs for Egyptian patients was to obtain relief from feelings of dependency and being a burden on the family. In contrast, American patients expressed a need for greater psychological support. The most commonly expressed attitude toward the diagnosis by the Egyptian patients was stoicism and fatalism, while among American patients it was to fight and adapt.[24]

Arab cancer patients have been reported to have very high levels of psychiatric distress and anxiety.[28] It has been suggested that religious faith, the provision of information, as well as family support and communication, are important factors that can help to mediate this distress.[24,29-31]

Pain

A particularly difficult issue for both patients and their families at the end of life is the experience of pain and other uncontrollable physiological symptoms such as incontinence. A number of studies have identified barriers to the treatment of pain at the end of life, or for conditions such as cancer. These include cultural attitudes regarding the use of narcotic medications which leads to the limited availability of narcotics, the undertreatment of pain due to fears of addiction, and tensions between different healthcare providers.[32,33]

A study of pediatric cancer pain from Jordan reported that the prevalence of pain in this population was very high, and was undertreated. The parents of the children did not express concerns about the use of narcotics for their children's pain. Rather, their focus was on obtaining pain relief for their children by whatever means possible. In addition, the study highlighted the strongly collective ethos of these families. The Western researchers were surprised to find that in trying to elicit parents' views about their prior personal experiences of physical pain, 19 out of the 22 parents interviewed stated that the worst pain that they had ever personally experienced was having a child diagnosed with cancer. This response persisted despite attempts by the researchers to probe further.[34] This reaction might indicate either the perception that it would be disloyal to change the focus from the patient to the parents' experience, or that indeed the pain of a family member is perceived so intensely that it metaphorically and psychologically erases the boundary between individuals. Research may be needed to clarify the significance of this finding.

A study from Morocco that also explored the issue of children's cancer pain found that cultural issues including fear of addiction were factors interfering with adequate treatment of pain in this population.[33]

In treating pain, particularly at the end of life, a proactive and organized approach should be strongly considered. Pain is frequently undertreated. For example, in the United States up to 50% of patients with severe persistent pain are inadequately treated.[35] Since pain is a subjective experience that is perceived only by the individual, patient assessment of the severity and quality of the pain is the best way to evaluate it. Cognitive, psychological and cultural factors all modify the experience and expression of pain, therefore, using a standardized scale (for example, ranking pain on a scale of 1–10) is often helpful. The health provider should remember that proactive and adequate treatment of pain reduces patient anxiety; reduced anxiety, in turn, often leads to much lower total analgesic needs.[36]

Medication is the foundation of pain management; use of the World Health Organization's medication ladder,[37] in which selection of the appropriate analgesic agent is based on the severity and type of pain experienced, is appropriate in almost all cases. Particularly in cancer pain, the provider should not hesitate to move to opioid management when needed; although addiction and abuse are frequent concerns for healthcare providers, the development of addiction in patients receiving narcotics for analgesia is actually quite uncommon.[37] A frequently observed manifestation of opioid-seeking behaviors in patients with pain is termed "pseudoaddiction". This condition is caused by the undertreatment of pain, and superficially resembles addictive behavior. It disappears with adequate pain treatment.[38]

The end of life

End-of-life decisions are difficult. Issues such as deciding to continue what may be futile care, or whether to withhold treatments or to withdraw care from terminally ill patients, are among the most ethically ambiguous and difficult that a health provider can make. Preferences for management of the end of life are strongly affected by culture. A study of a Lebanese intensive care unit found that decisions regarding the end of life were frequently made by medical personnel alone without family or patient involvement.[39] Another study that explored the process of deciding to withhold or withdraw life-sustaining treatments from neonates found that only rarely did parents want to be involved in the decision to withhold or terminate futile care. Most frequently, the parents would acquiesce silently when withdrawal was proposed, but would not explicitly articulate their agreement.[40]

TABLE 10.1 Guidelines for health providers at the end of life[41]

- Conduct frequent meetings with the patient and/or family in a quiet private area.
- Conduct a thorough assessment of religious and cultural beliefs.
- Use appropriate language (no medical jargon) to improve understanding.
- Prepare the family to see the patient, particularly if there are major physical or mental changes that may have occurred since the patient was last seen by family.
- Allow the patient and family private time as needed.

A model for dealing with end-of-life issues has been developed by researchers at the American University of Beirut Medical Center. They focused on the process of enhancing end-of-life care through interventions that included improving communication between the family, medical providers and, when necessary, the hospital ethics committee. Interestingly, it was found that communication between medical personnel was a key issue that needed to be addressed in this situation. This is not surprising, given the importance of presenting the family with clear and cohesive recommendations about further care.[41] Some of their guidelines for improving communication at the end of life are summarized in Table 10.1.

Conclusion

It has been said that, rather than being an evil, death is the essential condition for life. With this in mind, it is important to ensure that we place the same emphasis on providing high-quality care for those who are dying and their families as we do for other patients. Understanding patient and family worries, and giving these the same priority as other medical issues, is important even when we do not have more to offer them.

References

1 Granqvist HN. *Muslim Death and Burial: Arab customs and traditions studied in a village in Jordan.* Helsinki; 1965.

2 Racy J. Death in an Arab culture. *Ann N Y Acad Sci* 1969; **164 (3):** 871–80.

3 Errihani H, Abarrou N, Ayemou A *et al.* Psychosocial characteristics of Moroccan cancer patients: a survey of 1000 cases from the National Oncology Institute of Rabat. *Revue Francophone de Psycho-Oncologie* 2005; **4 (2):** 80–5.

4 Sibai AM, Fletcher A, Hills M *et al.* Non-communicable disease mortality rates using the verbal autopsy in a cohort of middle aged and older populations in Beirut during wartime, 1983–93. *J Epidemiol Community Health* 2001; **55 (4):** 271–6.

5 Sibai AM, Nuwayhid I, Beydoun M *et al.* Inadequacies of death certification in Beirut: who is responsible? *Bull World Health Organ* 2002; **80 (7):** 555–61.

6 Ruhnke GW, Wilson SR, Akamatsu T *et al.* Ethical decision making and patient autonomy: a comparison of physicians and patients in Japan and the United States. *Chest* 2000; **118 (4):** 1172–82.

7 Gabbay BB, Matsumura S, Etzioni S *et al.* Negotiating end-of-life decision making: a comparison of Japanese and US residents' approaches. *Acad Med* 2005; **80 (7):** 617–21.

8 Swinbanks D. Medical ethics: Japanese doctors keep quiet. *Nature* 1989; **339 (6225):** 409.

9 Feldman MD, Zhang J, Cummings SR. Chinese and US internists adhere to different ethical standards. *J Gen Intern Med* 1999; **14 (8):** 469–73.

10 Bruera E, Neumann CM, Mazzocato C *et al.* Attitudes and beliefs of palliative care physicians regarding communication with terminally ill cancer patients. *Palliat Med* 2000; **14 (4):** 287–98.

11 Baile WF, Lenzi R, Parker PA *et al.* Oncologists' attitudes toward and practices in giving bad news: an exploratory study. *J Clin Oncol* 2002; **20 (8):** 2189–96.

12 Hamadeh GN, Adib SM. Cancer truth disclosure by Lebanese doctors. *Soc Sci Med* 1998; **47 (9):** 1289–94.

13 Qasem AA, Ashour TH, Al-Abdulrazzaq HK *et al.* Disclosure of cancer diagnosis and prognosis by physicians in Kuwait. *Int J Clin Pract* 2002; **56 (3):** 215–18.

14 Mobeireek AF, al-Kassimi FA, al-Majid SA *et al.* Communication with the seriously ill: physicians' attitudes in Saudi Arabia. *J Med Ethics* 1996; **22 (5):** 282–5.

15 Harrison A, al-Saadi AM, al-Kaabi AS *et al.* Should doctors inform terminally ill patients? The opinions of nationals and doctors in the United Arab Emirates. *J Med Ethics* 1997; **23 (2):** 101–7.

16 Adib SM, Hamadeh GN. Attitudes of the Lebanese public regarding disclosure of serious illness. *J Med Ethics* 1999; **25 (5):** 399–403.

17 Bedikan A, Thompson S. Saudi community attitude toward cancer. *Annals of Saudi Medicine* 1985; **3:** 161–6.

18 Duffy SA, Jackson FC, Schim SM *et al.* Racial/ethnic preferences, sex preferences, and perceived discrimination related to end-of-life care. *J Am Geriatr Soc* 2006; **54 (1):** 150–7.

19 Buckman R, Kason Y. *How to Break Bad News: a guide for health care professionals.* Baltimore: Johns Hopkins University Press; 1992.

20 Freedman B. Offering truth: one ethical approach to the uninformed cancer patient. *Arch Intern Med* 1993; **153 (5):** 572–6.

21 Harris JJ, Shao J, Sugarman J. Disclosure of cancer diagnosis and prognosis in Northern Tanzania. *Soc Sci Med* 2003; **56 (5):** 905–13.

22 Klitzman R. Complications of culture in obtaining informed consent. *Am J Bioeth* 2006; **6 (1):** 20–1; discussion W27–8.

23 Gordon DR, Paci E. Disclosure practices and cultural narratives: understanding concealment and silence around cancer in Tuscany, Italy. *Soc Sci Med* 1997; **44 (10):** 1433–52.

24 Ali NS, Khalil HZ, Yousef W. A comparison of American and Egyptian cancer patients' attitudes and unmet needs. *Cancer Nurs* 1993; **16 (3):** 193–203.

25 Al-Shahri MZ. Culturally sensitive caring for Saudi patients. *J Transcult Nurs* 2002; **13 (2):** 133–8.

26 Al-Shahri MZ, al-Khenaizan A. Palliative care for Muslim patients. *J Support Oncol* 2005; **3 (6):** 432–6.

27 Sarhill N, LeGrand S, Islambouli R *et al.* The terminally ill Muslim: death and dying from the Muslim perspective. *Am J Hosp Palliat Care* 2001; **18 (4):** 251–5.

28 Khatib J, Salhi R, Awad G. Distress in cancer patients in KHCC: a study using the Arabic-modified version of distress thermometer in the King Hussein Cancer Center. *Arab Journal of Psychiatry* 2003; **14 (2):** 106–15.

29 Ali NS, Khalil HZ. Identification of stressors, level of stress, coping strategies, and coping effectiveness among Egyptian mastectomy patients. *Cancer Nurs* 1991; **14 (5):** 232–9.

30 Ali NS, Khalil HZ. Effect of psychoeducational intervention on anxiety among Egyptian bladder cancer patients. *Cancer Nurs* 1989; **12 (4):** 236–42.

31 Eapen V, Revesz T. Psychosocial correlates of paediatric cancer in the United Arab Emirates. *Support Care Cancer* 2003; **11 (3):** 185–9.

32 Abu-Saad H. Cultural group indicators of pain in children. *Matern Child Nurs J* 1984; **13 (3):** 187–96.

33 McCarthy P, Chammas G, Wilimas J *et al.* Managing children's cancer pain in Morocco. *J Nurs Scholarsh* 2004; **36 (1):** 11–15.

34 Forgeron PA, Finley GA, Arnaout M. Pediatric pain prevalence and parents' attitudes at a cancer hospital in Jordan. *J Pain Symptom Manage* 2006; **31 (5):** 440–8.

35 The management of persistent pain in older persons. *J Am Geriatr Soc* 2002; **50 (6 Suppl):** S205–24.

36 Cascinu S, Giordani P, Agostinelli R *et al.* Pain and its treatment in hospitalized patients with metastatic cancer. *Support Care Cancer* 2003; **11 (9):** 587–92.

37 Bope ET, Douglass AB, Gibovsky A *et al.* Pain management by the family physician: the family practice pain education project. *J Am Board Fam Pract* 2004; **17 Suppl:** S1–12.

38 Douglass A. Pain. In: Rakel R, Bope E, editors. *Conn's Current Therapy.* Philadelphia: Saunders Elsevier; 2007. p. 3.

39 Yazigi A, Riachi M, Dabbar G. Withholding and withdrawal of life-sustaining treatment in a Lebanese intensive care unit: a prospective observational study. *Intensive Care Med* 2005; **31 (4):** 562–7.

40 Da Costa D, Ghazal H, Al-Khusaibi S. "Do Not Resuscitate" orders and ethical decisions in a neonatal intensive care unit in a Muslim community. *Arch Dis Child Fetal Neonatal Ed* 2002; **86:** F115–119.

41 Gebara J, Tashjian H. End-of-life practices at a Lebanese hospital: courage or knowledge? *J Transcult Nurs* 2006; **17 (4):** 381–8.

PART 3

Mental health

CHAPTER 11

Approach to the patient in primary care psychiatry

(* *Laeth S Nasir and Arwa K Abdul-Haq*

Introduction

International studies suggest that 30% of patients who are seen in the primary care setting have a diagnosable psychiatric disorder, and that an equal number suffer from significant psychological distress that warrants careful follow-up.[1] Many studies have focused on the under-recognition and under-treatment of patients with psychological disorders in primary care practice throughout the world. Contributing factors are reported to include physician-related factors, such as deficient skills in interview and diagnosis, competing clinical priorities leading to preferential focus on physical problems, and the lack of available resources for treatment and follow-up. Other factors have not been well researched, but may be particularly relevant in the Arab world. These may include perceptions that the physician maintains patient dignity and allows them to save face if the diagnosis of a "shameful" condition such as depression is concealed.[2]

While the development of classification and standardized diagnostic systems such as the *Diagnostic and Statistical Manual of Mental Disorders*, 4th edition (DSM-IV), and *International Classification of Diseases*, version 10 (ICD-10), have greatly improved the reliability and reproducibility of psychiatric diagnoses, particularly for research purposes, they are often not a good fit for primary care, in which patients often present with multiple diagnoses and undifferentiated disorders frequently classified under the "not otherwise specified" or "subthreshold" DSM or ICD categories.[3] This suggests to health providers that these diagnoses are not clinically important. Providers are also left with little guidance regarding preferred treatment of these problems, despite the fact that in primary care studies, subthreshold disorders result in nearly as much disability as "categorizable" psychiatric disorders.[4] Not uncommonly, symptoms will wax and wane over time, so that at times patients will meet criteria for a psychiatric disorder, but not at other times, regardless of treatment.

The picture is further complicated by the fact that much of the information available in the region comes from studies of psychiatric populations. Therefore, data from these studies may have limited relevance in the primary care setting. This may lead to discrepancies between the presentation and classification of disease as described in the available literature, and what is observed clinically in the Arab world. Conceptualization of disease categories and symptom recognition in psychiatry are shaped to a large extent by the cultural norms and values of the societies where the classification systems were developed. There is a real need to explore different symptom patterns and diagnostic criteria in order to more accurately describe the presentation of psychiatric disorders in primary care in Arab countries.

Primary care psychiatry in the Arab world

As is the case in most of the world, psychiatric disorders have been reported to be associated with a great deal of stigma in Arab countries.[5-7] Psychiatric issues are seen by many as social or moral issues, rather than medical problems, to be dealt with through family, religious and social avenues. Disordered behavior or affect violates societal expectations of proper conduct, and is often perceived to reflect poorly on the patients' family of origin. Studies carried out in the Arab world and other developing countries suggest that individuals suffering from psychosocial problems may first seek attention through the extended family. If this proves insufficient, help may be sought from traditional or folk healers.[8] Only after these avenues are exhausted will the sufferer present to a physician or psychiatrist. Anecdotally, the patients' and families' perception of stigma increases when a formal psychiatric diagnosis is made. Few studies exist that explore the harmful effects of stigma due to psychiatric illness on patients and their families.[9]

Some individuals believe that mental illness is due to sorcery and other supernatural forces. This tends to be more common in older and less educated populations.[10-13] One study reports that the prevalence of these beliefs is independent of educational level.[14] Tactfully exploring the belief system of the patient and family is important. An understanding of the patient's illness model will facilitate the clinician's ability to frame the problem, and subsequently make it intelligible and credible to the patient and family. In devout patients, incorporation of religious explanations and practices into the healing process is often helpful.

Screening for psychiatric disorders

Individuals may experience difficulty in articulating details of their emotional state due to social expectations that they suppress expressions of intrapsychic and interpersonal conflict. Among many patients, the prospect of suffering from a mental illness elicits feelings of dread because they fear being ostracized by family and community. This can make screening for and treatment of mental illness a difficult undertaking for the primary care physician. One non-threatening and sensitive but non-specific screening test for the presence of psychosocial problems is to ask: "How is your sleep?" A reply indicating problems should prompt the clinician to explore symptoms of depression, anxiety and psychosocial stressors. Because metaphors and expressions of distress differ from community to community, physicians should make an effort to recognize colloquialisms and idiosyncratic presentations that represent psychological distress in their own patient population and local culture. Some signs of psychiatric distress, such as irritability or withdrawal from social activities, may not be reported by patients themselves but are often elicited from accompanying friends or relatives.

The use of self-report "pencil and paper" screening tests for psychiatric problems has not been studied in Arab countries. It is likely that these would not be well accepted by patients; where many people place great value on human contact and communication, they may feel neglected or vulnerable if they are expected to complete a form that asks about their emotional state.

Presentation of psychiatric problems

In the primary care setting, psychiatric problems usually present subtly. Most patients who present with psychosocial problems are unable to make sense of their confusing mixture of symptoms. Just as many patients suffering from angina complain of heartburn or arm pain, many people misattribute their psychological symptoms and tend to describe them in more familiar (therefore physical) terms. Somatic symptoms may also serve as a form of communication that allows the sufferer to obtain support or as a covert negotiating strategy in conflicts with their family or others. However, this does not necessarily mean that the symptoms are intentional, willfully produced or conscious. In most cases, individuals are unaware of the motivations that perpetuate the symptoms.

Vague, recurrent symptoms, such as chest tightness, dizziness or fatigue, are encountered most often in the primary care setting. Listening carefully to the patient frequently provides clues in the form of associated affective symptoms. In Western studies, frequent clinic attenders tend to have a high incidence of psychiatric disorders. This also seems to be true from clinical experience in Arab countries.

A dramatic presentation may be seen in patients who present with conversion or dissociative symptoms, often in an emergent setting. These patients tend to be younger, female and less educated; they often present with loss of consciousness, pseudoseizures, sensory loss or mutism.[15,16] Although such presentations may mislead clinicians initially, careful history-taking will often uncover an initially unsuspected psychiatric disorder. Depression, anxiety and personality disorders may be observed in these individuals.

Interviewing the patient with a suspected psychiatric disorder in primary care

In the primary care setting, dealing with most psychiatric problems is a process that involves two major steps. The first is making a diagnosis. This involves sorting through the patient's various symptoms and understanding the place and prominence that they occupy in the patient's life. The second part is to negotiate successfully with the patient (and often the family) regarding treatment.

The primary care setting has unique features that may both hinder and facilitate the detection and treatment of psychiatric problems. Factors that interfere with diagnosis include time pressure, the reluctance of the patient to reveal sensitive aspects of his or her illness, lack of privacy and competing clinical demands.

One of the major differences between primary care and psychiatric populations is the fact that virtually all patients and their families who present to psychiatric settings have already accepted a psychiatric dimension to their illness. On the other hand, in primary care settings, this is seldom the case. Patients with psychological problems tend to present a physical symptom or symptoms as a "ticket of admission" because of the conscious or unconscious perception that physical symptoms are a more acceptable reason to see to the physician. It is not uncommon for patients to have no awareness that they are suffering from a psychiatric problem. Others may suspect that they are suffering from a psychiatric problem but consciously or unconsciously resist the diagnosis. Some of these patients visit the health provider to obtain a provisional physical diagnosis. This provides some short-term reassurance that their problem is "not psychological". Detecting psychiatric problems in these settings can be challenging, particularly when other clinical problems are simultaneously offered. Studies have demonstrated that the more physical symptoms a patient presents in the clinical encounter, the less likely it is that the clinician will make a psychiatric diagnosis.[3]

Time pressure reduces the ability of the provider to gather sufficient information to formulate a differential diagnosis. It also inhibits the development of a trusting relationship through which a diagnosis can be negotiated, and from which a mutually acceptable plan of treatment can arise.

Structure of the primary care visit

Strengths of the primary care setting include the opportunity to develop an ongoing relationship with the patient, knowledge of his or her general health and social circumstances, and the ability to develop an impression of patient and family coping styles. Although the traditional "acute care" model of medical care continues to be the worldwide standard for clinical visits, where evaluation, diagnosis and treatment of problems occur within the same visit, a more appropriate model for chronic problems in primary care may be one that involves ongoing longitudinal care.

In dealing with psychiatric problems, where evaluation and diagnosis can seldom be neatly structured to fit into a single clinic visit, this longitudinal care concept can be used to the clinician's advantage. Consequently, the evaluation and treatment of many psychosocial problems may be allowed to unfold over several visits. For example, if the clinician asks the patient to observe how stress and fatigue affects his or her symptoms early in the process, a psychological dimension can be gradually introduced into the picture. This is particularly useful in those who are perceived to be resistant to a psychological explanation for their symptoms. Presenting the possibility in an indirect fashion will allow the patient and family time to reflect on the relative physical and psychological contributions of the illness. For this technique to be effective, it is important for the clinician to maintain a non-judgmental, respectful and focused attitude toward all the patient's problems.

For example, the clinician might say: "I'm not sure what this symptom represents at this time. Possibly it could be _____ (a physical condition). I would like you to try this medicine. Remember, any symptom may be made worse by stress. I want you to monitor your condition over the next few days and tell me whether things are a little worse when you are tired or stressed."

Another technique involves sharing the differential diagnosis with the patient, including both physical and psychological entities. If testing or a therapeutic trial for possible physical problems is unproductive, the patient will often return to the next visit more willing to consider the psychosocial dimensions of the problem.

Formulating a psychiatric diagnosis

When obtaining and synthesizing information from a patient with a psychiatric problem, it is useful to consider the history from several complementary perspectives: the biological, social and psychological. Biological factors include the presence of genetic predisposition to psychiatric disorders, such as a family or personal history of depression, bipolar disorder or schizophrenia, the presence of an intercurrent illness or medication, or alcohol or drug use. Psychological factors relate to habitual cognitive patterns or thinking styles. Examples include excessive pessimism, self-blame or catastrophic thinking. Social factors include problematic relationships, spousal or child abuse, employment problems, or other variables that may be present. A careful history will help to clarify the relative contribution of each of these factors to the clinical picture.

Another important issue is evaluating the degree of suffering and dysfunction the symptom or symptoms are causing. What consequences do the symptoms have for the patient and/or his or her family? Examples include disturbed social interactions, inability to fulfill expected social or occupational roles, or emotional suffering.

Gaining a good understanding of the patient's problem from the patient's own point of view is just as important as gathering and synthesizing the information needed to make a differential diagnosis. Allowing the patient some time to speak and demonstrating understanding are often profoundly therapeutic for the patient, even if no further action is needed. Listening, acknowledgement, support and ongoing monitoring of patients' symptoms are all that is needed in many psychosocial problems presenting in this way. Understanding the patient's point of view creates an atmosphere of trust and cooperation in which the patient is then able to have the confidence that any solutions that may be offered by the health provider will be the right ones. Conversely, if the patient's concerns, both revealed and concealed, are not addressed, acceptance of the diagnosis and compliance with treatment are unlikely.[17] Establishing a mutual perspective with the patient requires a physician to reflect his or her understanding of the problem to the patient, using non-clinical language: "It sounds like you have been feeling sad and tired over the past two months. Is that right?" Sharing your understanding with the patient, and allowing him or her to respond and, if necessary, clarify your understanding is critical. Throughout the interview, while summarizing and reflecting the patient's story, look to the patient to give you non-verbal clues that you are on the right track. Examples of this might include nodding and smiling. If these non-verbal cues are not elicited, the clinician must consider that they are not addressing all of the patient's concerns or that they had inadvertently offended the patient in some way.

Frequently, in the primary care setting, by the end of the visit the clinician is still unclear as to whether a significant psychiatric condition exists or not. At this point, choices for further management include obtaining further information or studies, reassessment at a future visit, or referral to a mental health professional for further evaluation. Often, in cases that do not require immediate intervention and treatment, it is useful to see the patient back at an appropriate interval. It is not unusual for patients with mild or vague symptoms to return to a follow-up visit reporting resolution of their previous symptoms. Sometimes, they will present a new set of symptoms that may form a more readily recognizable pattern (*see* Table 11.1).

Involvement of others in the interview

In Arab culture, norms for the involvement of family and others in medical care are often different from those in other parts of the world where individualism is emphasized. Therefore, it is not unusual for patients to present to the medical visit with friends or family. This transforms the "standard" classically described dyadic doctor–patient relationship of the Western medical literature into a triadic one, comprising patient, family and physician.

Studies of triadic medical encounters from other parts of the world suggest that the presence of a third individual in the medical visit changes the dynamics of the clinical encounter in important ways.[18] These may include loss of intimacy between physician and patient, the formation of coalitions, contention and decreased patient participation.[19] Some researchers have suggested that companions assume one of three roles in the encounter: as advocate, passive participant, or antagonist.[20] Others report that the companion may sometimes behave as a "hidden patient"; having needs of their own to be addressed.[21] A study from Japan reported that the companion may serve an important role as "patient facilitator" or spokesman, and that this role was more pronounced with increased patient debility.[22] It is interesting to note that the available literature consists almost exclusively of either parents and their minor children, or elderly people and their caregivers. This tends to confirm the clinical observation that, in other regions, companions tend to present with those at the extremes of age, while in Arab countries, it is not uncommon for people of any age to present with a companion.

Implications of this pattern for the clinical visit and outcomes have not been well studied in the Arab world. It might be hypothesized that the frequency with which patients present with companions to the medical encounter is due to perceptions of familial obligation, loyalty or solidarity. It may be that concerns regarding confidentiality are less important; an individual's sickness is seen as a communal problem that is presented to the physician who is expected to be a resource for the group as much as for the individual patient. These hypotheses and others will need to be explored in clinical studies.

Our own approach to the presence of a companion is to use it as an opportunity to enrich our understanding of the patient's situation, and to attempt to enlist the companion as an ally to reinforce our treatment recommendations. The first task is to identify and try to clarify the role of the person who accompanies the patient to the interview. We do not automatically assume that the patient companion is a family member, or even that the patient welcomes their presence in the interview. Asking the patient in the presence of the relative or friend whether she minds if the companion attends the consultation is almost never a good idea. Rather, clarifying the role of the companion directly, and excluding them from at least part of the interview should be considered, based on the specific situation. Most of the time, the presence of the companion is helpful, particularly in helping the patient to remember treatment recommendations and in helping the clinician to detect and understand interpersonal factors that might affect treatment.

Family involvement in the diagnosis

The clinician's ability to make the diagnosis of a psychiatric condition and proceed with treatment may be both enhanced and impeded by family involvement. The family can be the cause of the patient's distress, a major source of support, and sometimes both. From the clinician's perspective, having an observer who can provide additional background or corroborate reported symptoms such as irritability, withdrawal or even psychotic manifestations can be helpful, even critical, to making the diagnosis. On the other hand, family monitoring of patient–physician communication may inhibit a frank discussion of issues. Sometimes, but not always, this can be inferred by observing the patient's body language during the interview. One technique to keep the family feeling that they are involved while maintaining patient confidentiality is for the clinician to reverse the usual pattern of history-taking, and obtain a history from the observer's point of view first. Then, after reassuring the family member that they are an integral part of treatment, he or she is excused from the examining room, and the patient is asked for their perspective, including affective symptoms and possibly other information that the patient might have been reluctant to share.

TABLE 11. 1 A model for management of psychiatric disorders in the primary care setting

PRESENTATION	MANAGEMENT OPTIONS	EXAMPLES
Danger to self or others	Immediate evaluation and management, emergent referral if necessary	Psychoses (e.g. schizophrenia, bipolar disorder) Suicidal
Clear diagnosis	Targeted treatment. May or may not need referral, depending on clinician's expertise and available resources	Major depression Anxiety Adjustment disorder Substance abuse
Unclear diagnosis	Stepwise diagnostic testing, and trials of therapy if warranted. Alternatively, close observation without further evaluation, or referral if severe symptoms present	Chronic fatigue Unclear somatic symptoms

Not infrequently, patients and families are in denial regarding the nature of the illness. Often, a psychiatric explanation will be rejected, partly because of the perceived stigma and potential damage to the patient's or the family's reputation. The provider must be very alert to this response; etiquette will often prevent the patient or family from openly expressing disagreement with the physician's views. Instead, the patient may not comply with treatment, or will seek care elsewhere. One way to assess the degree of understanding and acceptance is to encourage the patient, at or near the end of the visit, to summarize his or her understanding of the diagnosis or treatment. Sometimes, acceptance of the diagnosis by key family members may be as important as, or more important than, getting the patient to accept the diagnosis. In these cases, having a close working knowledge and relationship with the family is critical. In most cases, it is important to involve family members in order to provide support, reassurance and education.[23]

In some situations, useful clinical information can be gleaned from the number and demeanor of accompanying family members. Habitual family patterns of behavior that may be contributing to the problem, such as demeaning, belittling or fighting, may be observed. Some clinicians report anecdotally that the larger the number of friends or family accompanying the patient, the more likely it is that the problem is a psychosocial one.

Integrating brief therapy into primary care

Managing patients who present with psychiatric conditions requires that the primary care physician be familiar with and proficient in all effective therapies that can be helpful to these patients. Therapy and counseling, although often practiced informally by physicians, has been traditionally viewed to be a separate discipline and outside the realm of the primary provider, for many reasons. One of the most important of these reasons is the perception that counseling is time-consuming and of questionable efficacy. Also, until recently, "counseling" was a vague term and meant little more than "talk" to allow patients to vent, and for the provider to give support and a bit of advice. Physicians often did this briefly, informally and intuitively without expecting much in terms of measurable improvement. Abundant evidence is now available that the efficacy of certain forms of therapy in the treatment of general psychological distress and several formal psychiatric disorders is comparable to that of medications.[24-9] When used in conjunction with pharmaceutical agents, counseling has been shown to augment their efficacy and produce a more sustained symptom resolution. More significantly for primary care physicians, some forms of therapy have been mainstreamed so they can be delivered briefly and concisely in the primary care setting. A brief, solution-focused therapy approach will be described to acquaint the reader with the principles of this practice and to demonstrate its applicability to the primary care setting.[30]

Theoretical background

Brief, solution-focused therapy is a model that is especially suited for working with individuals and families within societies where families are closely bonded and emotionally involved with each other. It also relies heavily on the patients' and families' views of the problem rather than depending on a theoretical ideology that may or may not be applicable to a particular cultural setting. These characteristics make solution-focused therapy a particularly attractive model for working with Arab patients.

The solution-focused model proposes that, in order to promote change and resolution of a problem, one should focus on two things: a vision of the situation in the problem-free state, and any change in current behavior that might move the person or the family out of the problem situation. In addition, the change made does not necessarily need to be directly related to the problem. Any change can prompt a cascade of changes that may improve the situation. *A detailed analysis of the nature or origin of the problem is not necessary or encouraged.*

Solution-focused therapy presumes that much distress experienced is due to patients' "getting stuck" in ineffective "false solutions" that they try over and over. By moving the patients' focus from the problem to the solution, people are helped to see beyond the problem; their former inability to see beyond the limited range of alternatives for effective solutions is replaced by a hopeful and optimistic outlook.

Practical approach

A few practical strategies and examples will be helpful to illustrate the use of this strategy in the primary care setting.

Assessment of the problem

The purpose of assessment is to get the patient's or the family's version of the problem. The patient is allowed to state his or her problem. If they offer a view or analysis of the origin or cause of the problem, this should be accepted. However, no more time should be spent on assessment of how the problem developed or is maintained. Instead, more information is sought about times and patterns of behavior when the problem did not exist or the "exceptions" – times when the problem was not there, or was even a little bit better.

A simple example of a clinical encounter of a patient presenting with "tiredness" might go something like this:

Physician:	When do you feel most tired?
Patient:	When I wake up in the morning.
Physician:	Are there any mornings when you don't feel tired?
Patient:	No, not really.
Physician:	Not even a little better?
Patient:	Yes, actually, I got up a few days ago and I felt a little better than usual.
Physician:	What was different about that morning?
Patient:	My brother was coming to town that day to visit.

These exceptions are highlighted and encouraged. In the above case, the patient was encouraged to try to call and see his brother more frequently, and intensify his social activities.

Sometimes it may be possible to create exceptions by changing a small detail of the problem. For example, if a wife feels most depressed or anxious during the day when she is at home by herself or with her small children, it could be suggested that when she gets up in the morning she should get dressed as though she were going out even if she is not intending to do so. This alone may produce enough change in her focus to interrupt the cycle of feelings of helplessness and hopelessness. In addition, time might be spent on assessment of future goals and defining and visualizing a problem-free state.

Questions that might be useful in assessment include:

•➤ What do you think is the problem?
•➤ How will you know the problem is solved?
•➤ How will you know you don't have to come here any more?
•➤ How will your feelings, thoughts and behavior be different?
•➤ How will other people be different?[31]

Therapeutic techniques

Three therapeutic techniques have been described as the mainstay of solution-focused therapy: the first is instructing the patient to think of things in his or her life that they would like to continue. This is a simple but very powerful question or assignment since it will redirect the patient's thoughts to what is going right rather than wrong in their lives. Answers may include things like hobbies, seeing certain friends or other activities. The second question involves having the patient focus on the times when the problem is not there or is a little better, and exploring the circumstances, feelings, thoughts and behaviors of the patient and related people during those times. This exercise will empower the patient to think of ways to recreate any of the circumstances to produce relief or improve the situation. The third element is often termed "the miracle question". The provider asks the patient: "If I could magically make the problem disappear, how would you know it?" "What would be different about your thoughts and your feelings?" Asking the patient to describe details of this state will reveal possibilities for change. This shift of perspective from the past to the future and from "problem talk" to "solution talk" proves to be self-enforcing most of the time, and results not only in problem resolution but in enhanced communication and an expanded, positive outlook. In the time-limited primary care setting, using these techniques to briefly obtain a view of the problem, focus on a small, incremental, behaviorally defined goal and on providing the patient with instructions for "homework" and follow-up is often highly effective and rewarding.

References

1 Üstün TB, Sartorius N. *Mental Illness in General Health Care: an international study.* Chichester; New York: Published on behalf of the World Health Organization [by] Wiley; 1995.
2 Nasir LS, Al-Qutob R. Barriers to the diagnosis and treatment of depression in Jordan: a nationwide qualitative study. *J Am Board Fam Pract* 2005; **18 (2):** 125–31.

3 Kirmayer LJ. Cultural variations in the clinical presentation of depression and anxiety: implications for diagnosis and treatment. *J Clin Psychiatry* 2001; **62 Suppl 13:** 22–8; discussion 29–30.

4 Sartorius N, Ustun TB, Costa e Silva JA *et al.* An international study of psychological problems in primary care: preliminary report from the World Health Organization Collaborative Project on Psychological Problems in General Health Care. *Arch Gen Psychiatry* 1993; **50 (10):** 819–24.

5 Al-Adawi S, Dorvlo AS, Al-Ismaily SS *et al.* Perception of and attitude towards mental illness in Oman. *Int J Soc Psychiatry* 2002; **48 (4):** 305–17.

6 Eapen V, Ghubash R. Help-seeking for mental health problems of children: preferences and attitudes in the United Arab Emirates. *Psychol Rep* 2004; **94 (2):** 663–7.

7 AbuMadini MS, Rahim SI. Psychiatric admission in a general hospital: patients' profile and patterns of service utilization over a decade. *Saudi Med J* 2002; **23 (1):** 44–50.

8 Al-Subaie A. Traditional healing experiences in patients attending a university outpatient clinic. *Arab Journal of Psychiatry* 1994; **5 (2):** 83–91.

9 Kadri N, Manoudi F, Berrada S *et al.* Stigma impact on Moroccan families of patients with schizophrenia. *Can J Psychiatry* 2004; **49 (9):** 625–9.

10 Alsugharyir M. Public view of the "evil eye" and its role in psychiatry. *Arab Journal of Psychiatry* 1996; **7 (2):** 152–60.

11 Ide BA, Sanli T. Health beliefs and behaviors of Saudi women. *Women's Health* 1992; **19 (1):** 97–113.

12 Fido A, Zahid MA. Coping with infertility among Kuwaiti women: cultural perspectives. *Int J Soc Psychiatry* 2004; **50 (4):** 294–300.

13 El-Islam MF. Cultural aspects of illness behavior. *Arab Journal of Psychiatry* 1995; **6 (1):** 13–18.

14 El-Islam MF, Malasi T. Delusions and education. *Journal of Operational Psychiatry* 1985; **16 (2):** 29–31.

15 Shunaigat W. Clinical characteristics of conversion disorder in Jordan. *Arab Journal of Psychiatry* 2001; **12 (1):** 38–44.

16 Al-Habeeb T, Abdulgani Y, Al-Ghamdi M *et al.* The sociodemographic and clinical pattern of hysteria in Saudi Arabia. *Arab Journal of Psychiatry* 1999; **10 (2).**

17 Cruz M, Pincus HA. Research on the influence that communication in psychiatric encounters has on treatment. *Psychiatr Serv* 2002; **53 (10):** 1253–65.

18 Coe R, Prendergast C. The formation of coalitions: interaction strategies in triads. *Sociology Health and Illness* 1985; **7 (2):** 236–47.

19 Beisecker AE. The influence of a companion on the doctor–elderly patient interaction. *Health Commun* 1989; **1 (1):** 55–70.

20 Adelman RD, Greene MG, Charon R. The physician–elderly patient–companion triad in the medical encounter: the development of a conceptual framework and research agenda. *Gerontologist* 1987; **27 (6):** 729–34.

21 Haug M. Elderly patients, caregivers and physicians: theory and research on health care triads. *Journal of Health and Social Behavior* 1994; **35 (1):** 1–12.

22 Ishikawa H, Roter DL, Yamazaki Y *et al.* Physician–elderly patient–companion communication and roles of companions in Japanese geriatric encounters. *Soc Sci Med* 2005; **60 (10):** 2307–20.

23 El-Islam MF. Some cultural aspects of the Arab patient–doctor relationship. *Bulletin of the Board of International Affairs of the Royal College of Psychiatrists* 2005; **7:** 18–20.

24 Milgrom J, Negri LM, Gemmill AW *et al.* A randomized controlled trial of psychological interventions for postnatal depression. *Br J Clin Psychol* 2005; **44 (Pt 4):** 529–42.

25 Young JF, Mufson L, Davies M. Efficacy of interpersonal psychotherapy–adolescent skills training: an indicated preventive intervention for depression. *J Child Psychol Psychiatry* 2006; **47 (12):** 1254–62.

26 Neugebauer R, Kline J, Bleiberg K *et al.* Preliminary open trial of interpersonal counseling for subsyndromal depression following miscarriage. *Depress Anxiety* 2007; **24 (3):** 219–22.

27 Schut HA, Stroebe MS, van den Bout J *et al.* Intervention for the bereaved: gender differences in the efficacy of two counselling programmes. *Br J Clin Psychol* 1997; **36 (Pt 1):** 63–72.

28 Wolf NJ, Hopko DR. Psychosocial and pharmacological interventions for depressed adults in primary care: a critical review. *Clin Psychol Rev* 2007.

29 McEvoy PM, Nathan P. Effectiveness of cognitive behavior therapy for diagnostically heterogeneous groups: a benchmarking study. *J Consult Clin Psychol* 2007; **75 (2):** 344–50.

30 De Shazer S, Dolan YM, Korman H. *More Than Miracles: the state of the art of solution-focused brief therapy.* New York: Haworth Press; 2007.

31 De Jong P, Berg IK. *Interviewing for Solutions.* 2nd ed. Pacific Grove, CA: Brooks/Cole; 2002.

CHAPTER 12

Anxiety and somatoform disorders

(* *Brigitte Khoury, Michel R Khoury and Laeth S Nasir*

Introduction

Anxiety is a normal and adaptive response that alerts individuals to danger, and as such, is a universal emotion. Normal anxiety typically occurs in response to an external stressor and terminates with the resolution of the stressor. Normal anxiety is also proportionate to the threat faced, and may be developmentally mediated. For example, while anxiety manifested by crying would be a normal response to parting from a parent in a toddler, this would be distinctly abnormal in a teenager. The level of anxiety experienced in an encounter with an insect should not be the same as that experienced when being attacked by a dog.

Anxiety disorders are a group of psychiatric disorders that share persistent anxiety that is more severe than expected, given the situation. The anxiety often results in significant levels of personal distress. Distinguishing between what constitutes normal from abnormal anxiety on the continuum of behavior can be difficult at times. When making this distinction, clinicians usually base their decisions on the perceived degree of distress that is reported by the individual, impairment in social and occupational functioning, and the appropriateness of the degree of anxiety with a given environmental cue.

Anxiety disorders are frequently co-morbid with another psychiatric disorder, such as major depressive disorder. Sometimes, particularly in the primary care setting, it is challenging to differentiate between the two. Often, both diagnoses are made since the patient presents with an array of traits and symptoms covering both disorders, necessitating a dual diagnosis. Co-existence of two psychiatric disorders might change the prognosis or outcome of the conditions. For example, studies from Western countries show that patients having co-morbid panic disorder (a type of anxiety disorder) and major depression have a particularly high rate of suicide. Sometimes individuals with an underlying psychotic disorder present with symptoms of anxiety, which is an appropriate physiological response to the hallucinations and/or delusions that they are experiencing. Therefore, clinicians should be alert to the detection of co-morbid psychiatric conditions.

Somatoform disorders are another type of anxiety disorder often encountered in the primary care setting. These disorders are characterized by the tendency of the patient to express psychological distress as physical symptoms. Often, patients with somatization will present with symptoms such as palpitations, frequent urination, fatigue, abdominal pain, nausea, headache or backache. Furthermore, some patients with anxiety or depression may have a multitude of these symptoms, or present in such a dramatic fashion that the clinician may feel quite overwhelmed. Authorities report that anxiety and mood disorders are often obscured by somatic symptoms in Arab patients;[1] this complicates the clinical presentation and makes it difficult for the physician to be able to identify them as psychiatric disorders.

Anxiety disorders

Anxiety disorders are classified into categories that reflect distinct subtypes based on their clinical manifestations. The *International Classification of Diseases* (ICD-10) published by the World Health Organization[2] and the American Psychiatric Association's *Diagnostic and Statistical Manual of Mental Disorders* 4th edition[3] have each established their own classifications for anxiety disorders and somatoform disorders. While the DSM-IV separates them in two different chapters, the ICD-10 joins them under one chapter titled: "Neurotic, stress-related and somatoform disorders."

In the DSM-IV, anxiety disorders are categorized as the following: specific phobia, social phobia, panic disorder with or without agoraphobia, generalized anxiety disorder (GAD), obsessive-compulsive disorder (OCD), acute stress disorder, and post-traumatic stress disorder (PTSD).

In the ICD-10, anxiety disorders are divided into the following categories: phobic anxiety disorders, agoraphobia, social phobias, specific phobias, panic disorder, generalized anxiety disorder, obsessive compulsive disorder, reaction to severe stress and adjustment disorders, acute stress reaction, post-traumatic stress disorder and adjustment disorders.

The most easily recognized anxiety disorders (and the ones that patients most frequently seek help for) are those that cause significant impairments in social or occupational functioning, such as panic disorders or obsessive-compulsive disorders. In contrast, individuals with conditions such as generalized anxiety disorders and social phobia are much less likely to seek treatment, or may seek it much later. This is partly due to adjustments patients and their families make over time to compensate for their symptoms.

One large-scale study reported a 12-month prevalence of "any anxiety disorder" in a national sample from Lebanon to be 11.2%; this rate is comparable to prevalence surveys carried out in Western populations.[4] The study showed that anxiety disorders in Lebanon are the most prevalent mental disorder (11.2%) and more prevalent than mood disorders (6.6%), impulse-control disorders (2.2%), and substance abuse disorders (1.3%). In this study, significant socio-demographic correlates of anxiety disorders included being female and single. Moreover, the study revealed that respondents who were exposed to multiple (two or more) war-related traumatic events had more severe symptoms. It is also important to note that, compared to data from Western populations, Lebanese individuals with mental disorders receive considerably less professional treatment, and pursue more "non-medical solutions"; for example seeking the advice of religious figures, herbalists and fortune-tellers. Two-thirds of patients presented their symptoms to health professionals in primary care or other general medical specialties, and only a very small proportion sought care from a mental health provider. Formal treatment was less commonly sought for anxiety disorders (6.5%) than for mood disorders (19.3%). It was also more common for women than men to seek help for anxiety disorders.

In data from Egypt, Okasha *et al.* reported that anxiety disorders were diagnosed in 36% of a sample of university students.[5] Another study from an outpatient psychiatric setting evaluated the symptomatology of 120 patients with anxiety. The most common symptoms reported were: worrying (82%), irritability (73%), free-floating anxiety (70%), depressed mood (65%), tiredness (64%), restlessness (63%), anergia (no or lack of energy), and psychomotor retardation (61%). Moreover, 30% of the sample was diagnosed with panic attacks, 35% with situational anxiety, and 37% with specific phobias. Differences in clinical manifestations of anxiety were reported to vary depending on factors such as the patients' educational level and living conditions.[6]

Generalized anxiety disorder (GAD)

Generalized anxiety disorder (GAD) is one of the most common anxiety disorders in the general population. However, because of its vague symptoms, it is seldom recognized in the primary care setting. Studies indicate that it is twice as common among women as it is among men. The majority of individuals suffering from GAD have an additional psychiatric disorder, such as social phobia, major depression, specific phobia or panic disorder. Studies from the West suggest that early adverse childhood experiences, particularly witnessing violence, are an important factor in the genesis of GAD.[7]

According to the DSM-IV and the ICD-10, GAD is characterized by "free-floating anxiety" (anxiety without any obvious precipitant or cause). This is diagnosed when an individual has excessive worry or anxiety every day or nearly every day for six months or longer, associated with several psychological and/ or physical symptoms of anxiety. These may include muscle tension, fatigue, complaints of poor memory, and sleep disorders. Three or more of the following symptoms need to be present: restlessness, getting tired easily, decreased concentration, irritability, increased muscle tension and disturbed sleep.

Often these patients will admit to chronic rumination about the future, anticipation of negative events, and an inability to relax. Frequently, sufferers will worry about matters relating to family, work, finances or health. They may report avoidance of television or newspapers because of the additional anxiety caused by bad news. Alternatively, some patients will compulsively follow news reports as they are convinced that something bad is going to happen, and since often something bad does happen, it tends to confirm and reinforce their anxiety feelings.

In a study investigating the level of death anxiety across several countries, Abdel-Khalek distributed the Templer Death Anxiety Scale in Spain and five Arab countries (Egypt, Kuwait, Qatar, Lebanon and Syria) to undergraduate students. He reported that mean levels of anxiety for the Spanish sample were lower than those of the Arab countries.[8] Another study that compared levels of anxiety between college students in the United States and Kuwait reported higher levels of anxiety among the Kuwaiti students.[9]

Specific phobias

Specific phobias are defined as prominent, unjustified, excessive and persistent fear cued by exposure or anticipated exposure to a specific object or situation. The DSM-IV and the ICD-10 divide the types of specific phobias into four categories:

- *situational type:* fear of a specific situation such as heights, closed spaces, driving or airplanes
- *natural environment type:* fear of storms, catastrophes, earthquakes or water
- *animal type:* fear of animals or insects such as spiders, snakes or dogs
- *blood injection/injury type:* fear of seeing blood or invasive medical procedures, fear of injections, blood tests or injuries.

Individuals with "simple" phobias have no impairment in other domains of function; their functioning depends on their ability to avoid the feared object or situation. It is common, however, for these individuals to suffer from a panic attack if faced with the object or situation which they fear. These patients typically only come to a physician's attention when the phobia interferes significantly with their social or occupational functioning.

Specific phobias were reported to be the most prevalent but least severe type of anxiety disorder in Lebanon.[4]

Social phobia

Individuals with social phobia have a marked and persistent fear of social situations (such as initiating a conversation, attending social functions, eating in public) or performance (public speaking, small group involvement, attending classes), where they feel that they may be under scrutiny from others. It is often associated with low self-esteem and fear of criticism. Frequently these patients avoid coming to medical attention, and may be brought in by family members. They often exhibit symptoms of autonomic arousal such as shakiness or tension, blushing, sweating, and tremulousness of the voice.

Most patients with social phobia have a long history of shyness, often dating to childhood. Some data suggest that there is a strong heritable component.[10] Sometimes the history dates back to a particularly humiliating event. Social phobia may worsen with time. Self-medication is common, with sufferers often resorting to substances such as alcohol to reduce their anxiety prior to social situations. Studies from Saudi Arabia suggest that co-morbid depression is common.[11,12] Individuals with social anxiety are often under-diagnosed. However, the clinician should remember that if the patient does not have interference in his or her social or occupational functioning, by definition, he or she does not have a "disorder". Arab culture plays a significant role in ameliorating the impact of this condition, wherein close individual support and protection available from family and friends helps to decrease or eliminate psychological distress in these individuals by facilitating many important social functions. For example, among people with social phobia, family assistance in meeting a potential spouse helps to compensate for their lack of social ability. Additionally, women with social anxiety are often perceived to be shy and gentle, which is appreciated and desired as a feminine trait within Arab culture. Hence their problem may go unnoticed until they are faced with more social obligations and demands, at which time they may decide to seek help.

Panic disorder

Panic attacks are characterized by periods of overwhelming anxiety and fear, which come on abruptly for no apparent reason. According to the DSM-IV, they need to include at least four of the following symptoms: chills or hot flushes, derealization (a feeling of detachment from reality) or depersonalization (a feeling of detachment from oneself), chest pain, feelings of choking, feelings of going crazy or losing control, feeling dizzy or faint, nausea, palpitations, fear of dying, trembling or shaking, shortness of breath, paresthesias and sweating.

The ICD-10, in its classification for panic disorder, lists similar symptoms as the DSM-IV.

Episodes of severe autonomic over-activity (palpitations, dizziness, shakiness) are the hallmark of panic disorder. Some may be triggered by environmental factors, such as exercise, but mostly they occur spontaneously. Patients have persistent concerns about the cause of the attacks and having future attacks. In essence, they "fear the fear".

If the episodes are untreated, many patients will begin to suffer from agoraphobia, or anxiety about being in places or situations from where escape might be difficult, or help unavailable. This may develop into a fear of leaving the house and such patients may spend all their time at home, unable to go out and risk having a panic attack. Sufferers will try to avoid crowds, will make sure to carry a cell phone at all times, and will often refuse to leave home without someone to accompany them. It has been reported that manifestations of agoraphobia among women are rare in many Arab countries, because it is very acceptable, and in some areas customary or mandatory, for women to move out of the house only with a husband or a chaperone.[13]

A cross-national study on the epidemiology of panic disorder in ten countries, including Lebanon, showed the rates of female sufferers to be higher than those of males, with the median age of onset to be in the mid-20s, and significant rates of co-morbid agoraphobia and depression. These results were consistent with those obtained from the other countries in the study.[14]

Obsessive-compulsive disorder (OCD)

Obsessive-compulsive disorder (OCD) is characterized by anxiety-provoking intrusive thoughts (obsessions) that are accompanied by repeated ritualistic behavior whose purpose is to lessen or eliminate the anxiety caused by these obsessions. Symptoms cause considerable distress, and preoccupations can pertain to the smallest details in one's life, causing interference with daily social and occupational functioning. Obsessive ideas frequently include contamination, dirt, diseases and germs, real or imagined trauma, oZr some type of frightening theme. Compulsions often relate to washing, cleaning, orderliness or checking behaviors. Although the individual with OCD recognizes that her or his obsessions and subsequent compulsions are a product of his or her own thinking, and do not make sense, she or he cannot stop them.

It has been noted that patients in Arab countries suffering from OCD often have obsessions around religious issues, hence the compulsive behaviors are frequently related to prayers or religious rituals.

Waswas is a culture-specific obsessive-compulsive syndrome among practicing Muslims; the term refers to the whispered promptings of the devil, and includes doubts about the completeness or correctness of ritual ablutions, and/or doubts about the validity or correctness of elements of prayer rituals. This may lead to distress and excessive involvement in these activities. However, it may not be seen as requiring medical intervention; rather, the behavior may be normalized and conceptualized as an honorable response to Satanic distractions.[15]

It has also been noted by some authors that obsessions may have a sexual content, which raises their guilt level, hence pushing them to more prayers and religious rituals in order to compensate for the "sinful, sexual thoughts".[16] This creates a vicious cycle of OCD rituals, whereby the individual obsesses about sexual matters, which then leads him or her to obsessions about religious matters as a way to "be forgiven" for his or her sinful thoughts.

The ICD-10 divides the OCD category into further subcategories: predominantly obsessional thoughts or ruminations, and predominantly compulsive acts. The predominantly obsessional thoughts or ruminations subcategory emphasizes the presence of obsessions in the presenting clinical picture, which can take the form of mental images, ideas or impulses which are always distressing to the patient. Sometimes this presents as an indecisive and endless consideration of alternatives, resulting in an inability to make decisions in one's daily life. In this category, the presence of compulsions is not essential for the diagnosis. The predominantly compulsive acts subcategory emphasizes the presence of compulsive acts concerned with cleaning, checking or orderliness.

The rates of OCD are quite similar across Western and non-Western countries, as indicated by cross-national studies. However, the meaning, manifestations and understanding of the concept of anxiety may vary from one culture to another. This is evident in an excerpt from a book chapter by I. Al-Issa and S. Oudji (1998).[16]

> "In a study conducted in Saudi Arabia, Mahgoub and Abdel-Hafeiz (1991) found that compulsions, doubts, thoughts, impulses, fears, and images, in descending order, were the most frequent forms of OCD. Body-washing and fear of contamination related to religious themes were frequent among patients. In a study in Egypt, Okasha, *et al.* (1994) found that the most common obsessive symptoms were related to religious themes and contamination (60% each), while rituals (68%) were the most common compulsions. Religious and sexual themes were the most prevalent among patients. In another study in Qatar, obsessive thoughts of harming oneself or others were attributed to impulses induced by the devil among female patients (El-Islam, 1994) These religious themes seem to be more frequent among Muslim OCD patients than among Hindu patients studied by Akhtar *et al.* (1975) and are almost absent among Western patients."

Post-traumatic stress disorder (PTSD)

Post-traumatic stress disorder (PTSD) arises as a response to a stressful event or situation of an exceptionally threatening or catastrophic nature that is likely to cause distress in anyone. According to the DSM-IV, the essential feature is the development of characteristic symptoms following exposure to an extreme traumatic stressor involving direct personal experience of an event which involves actual or threatened death or serious injury or any other threat to one's physical integrity. It can also arise by learning about an unexpected violent death or threat of death or injury to a family member or a person close to the individual. The response must involve intense fear, helplessness or horror. In a review of the literature on the psychosocial consequences of war on civilians, Karam elucidates the fact that the mental health effects of war have been shown to cut across all strata of civilians. They affect not only high-risk groups like refugees, but also journalists covering the war, peacekeepers, as well as the partners of those exposed to violence.[17]

Some examples of traumatic events are sexual aggression (rape, sexual abuse), wars, torture, natural disasters (earthquakes, hurricanes), accidents, witnessing violence, military combat, being taken hostage, being victim of a robbery or being diagnosed with a fatal illness. PTSD symptoms are characterized by episodes of reliving the trauma (flashbacks), nightmares, emotional numbing, detachment from others, avoidance of situations reminiscent of the trauma, hypervigilance, hyperarousal which is often accompanied by a startled reaction, and insomnia. The onset of PTSD can be from a few weeks to several months following the trauma; the symptoms must be present for at least one month and cause significant distress and impairment in social and occupational functioning. Literature from population surveys in both North America and the Arab world suggests that, although men tend to be exposed to higher levels of trauma and violence, PTSD is more prevalent among women.[18] Co-morbidity of PTSD with another psychiatric disorder is very high; other anxiety disorders, depression and substance abuse are common associations.

The consequences of PTSD can be very long lasting. In a study of Lebanese civilians exposed to a church explosion, 39% of the victims met the criteria for PTSD even after a lapse of one year following the traumatic event.[19] Some populations in the Arab world living in regions with high levels of violence and war can suffer from very high rates of PTSD. One study from Gaza reported that nearly 73% of a sample of 239 children aged from six to 11 years suffered from PTSD symptoms of at least mild intensity, while 41% had moderate or severe symptoms.[20] Data from North America suggest that symptoms of PTSD resulting from trauma that was experienced during childhood has particular characteristics. These include difficulty with affect regulation (most commonly, inability to control anger or frustration), increased somatization and self-harm behavior.[21]

(*See also* Chapter 13, Post-traumatic stress disorder).

Acute stress disorder

Acute stress disorder is characterized by an exposure to a traumatic event or experience involving intense horror, fear or helplessness. The event usually involves a threat of death and/or a serious threat to physical integrity. It may have happened to the person or to others around him or her. Three or more of these symptoms are experienced: loss of emotions or numbing, depersonalization, derealization, dissociative amnesia and diminished awareness of surroundings. The event is re-experienced as distressing memories, recurrent nightmares, flashbacks, hallucinations, illusions, hypervigilance, hyperarousal, and an avoidance of anything associated with the trauma. The timeframe in this diagnosis is crucial: these symptoms last between two days to four weeks. If they persist for longer than that, then a diagnosis of PTSD is more likely.

Anxiety disorder due to a medical condition or to a substance

Anxiety disorders may also occur secondary to another condition, such as a medical illness (e.g. hyperthyroidism or pheochromocytoma) or substance abuse. In the former case, anxiety is seen as a direct result of a pre-existing medical condition. There must be evidence of a medical condition from the history, clinical findings or laboratory tests. Therefore it is essential for the clinician to establish the presence of a general medical condition and that the anxiety symptoms are etiologically related to it. In the case of substance-induced anxiety, the anxiety disorder is judged to be the direct physiological effect of a substance such as medication, drugs or alcohol. Therefore, a careful history should be taken to detect the intake of licit or illicit substances, including prescribed medications or caffeine, which may result in anxiety symptoms.

Conversely, substance abuse may occur as the result of attempts by a patient to self-medicate in the context of a pre-existing anxiety disorder. Even though the prevalence of anxiety in Lebanon is similar to that of other Western countries, the extent of benzodiazepine abuse is much higher.[22] Furthermore, in a co-morbidity study of substance abuse and psychiatric disorders done at St George's Hospital in Beirut, Lebanon, the rate of tranquilizer abuse was found to be the highest among patients with anxiety disorders; moreover, alcohol was also commonly abused.[23]

Somatoform disorders

The main characteristic of somatoform disorders is the presence of physical symptoms suggesting a medical condition, yet they are not medically explicable. The disorders cause significant distress, hence affecting occupational and social functioning. The physical symptoms are unintentional and involuntary and patients actually feel the pains and other sensations accompanying these symptoms. These disorders are often found in clinical settings, and patients suffering from them usually consult many physicians and undergo multiple tests and treatments, despite reassurance, before being referred for psychiatric treatment. If any physical disorders do exist, they do not explain the nature and magnitude of the symptoms reported by the patient, nor the level of distress and preoccupation.

The prominence of somatic expression of psychiatric disorders in many Arab countries is well documented in the literature.[24] One study sought to explain the high prevalence of somatized mental disorder (SMD) compared to psychologized mental disorders (PMD) and the notion that somatization is a metaphor to convey psychological distress. "Somatization is hypothesized to be an expression of personal and social distress in the form of bodily complaints with medical help-seeking. It is regarded as an adaptive mechanism for lessening psychic pain and changing it to physical pains for which there are treatments."[25] It has been hypothesized that by playing the sick role, patients obtain secondary gain through relief from their occupational and societal obligations, and by escaping the stigma attached to mental illness.[26] Females tend to be diagnosed with somatoform disorder more often than males.[27]

In the DSM-IV, somatoform disorders are divided into the following categories: somatization disorder, undifferentiated somatoform disorder, conversion disorder, pain disorder, hypochondriasis, and body dysmorphic disorder. The ICD-10 also includes a classification for somatoform disorders.

Somatization disorder

This disorder is characterized by physical symptoms that occur over many years involving different areas in the body, usually starting before age 30. Symptoms are not false, but really felt by the patient. He or she may describe symptoms in dramatic and emotional terms, seek care from more than one physician at the same time, describe symptoms in vague terms, and have complaints that medical tests fail to support.

Each of the following categories of symptoms must be present in order to diagnose the disorder:
- *4 pain symptoms:* pain related to at least four different sites in the body which includes headache, backache, stomach ache, joint pain and chest pain
- *2 gastrointestinal symptoms:* such as nausea, vomiting, diarrhea and bloating
- *1 sexual symptom:* such as erectile dysfunction, problems with menstruation, or sexual indifference.
- *1 pseudoneurological symptom:* such as problems with coordination or balance, paralysis, numbness, weakness, vision problems, hearing problems, seizures, difficulty swallowing, or urinary retention.

It is generally advisable to screen the patient initially for depression and anxiety, which often accompanies somatization disorder. A correct diagnosis can help to prevent unnecessary medical investigation. This disorder is also known as "hysteria" or "Briquet's syndrome". It is important for the clinician to remember that somatizing patients can also develop physical illnesses. Therefore, a previous diagnosis of somatization or hysteria does not rule out other medical problems. This often makes evaluation of these patients a challenge.

Undifferentiated somatoform disorder

The main feature of this disorder is one or more physical complaints which have persisted for six months or longer. Some of these symptoms can be fatigue, loss of appetite, gastrointestinal or urinary complaints. These symptoms cannot be explained by any medical condition or the effect of any substance and cause significant distress and interference in the patient's daily life. These symptoms may be used as "idioms of distress" to express personal and social problems, which the person is unable either to face or to express verbally. It is mostly seen in women from low socioeconomic backgrounds with limited education, and who resort to this means of communication to express their mental distress. This disorder has been called "neurasthenia" in different parts of the world.

Conversion disorder

The essential characteristic of this disorder is the presence of symptoms or deficits affecting motor or sensory function that suggest a neurological or medical condition, such as paralysis, blindness, deafness, loss of function in one limb or part of the body. Symptoms are usually preceded by conflicts or stressors; hence they are seen as a reaction to psychological pressures. The symptoms cannot be explained medically, cause significant distress and affect functioning.

Conversion disorder is seen as a symbolic resolution of a psychological conflict and is used to reduce the anxiety associated with such a conflict. Hence attention is focused on the physical symptom rather than on the real problem. Sometimes patients derive a "secondary gain" from this disorder, such as attention from family, or reduction of their work responsibilities or home chores due to the "illness". Although the individual may derive secondary gain, the symptoms, however, are neither feigned nor intentionally produced but rather felt very vividly by the sufferer.

Two independent authors studied the sociodemographic and clinical parameters of patients with conversion disorder in Saudi Arabia and Jordan, respectively.[27,28] Both studies showed that the majority of patients were single young women. Most of the patients presented with a single symptom, such as aphonia (inability to verbalize), fitlike movements (seizure-like or pseudo-seizure), loss of consciousness, decreased sensation and hyperventilation. The former study reported co-morbid clinical depression in 23.5% of patients. The latter study also identified psychosocial stressors to be present in 85% of patients; additionally, 58% of cases had concurrent psychiatric disorders, most commonly, depression and personality disorders. A study from Qatar reported similar findings and explored the role of social factors in precipitating the symptoms.[29] Psychiatric co-morbidity should always be sought in these patients due to the high levels of associated problems in this population.

Case vignette

A middle-aged man was brought into the emergency room on the stretcher seeming to be in and out of consciousness with his body half-paralyzed and something "wrong" in his chest area. The medical student on call started zealously calling his seniors and demanding the nurses to dial the cardiac team to resuscitate this man. However, the team took their time and did not respond to the urgency of the medical student. That was his first encounter with conversion disorder, whereby an individual seems to be having neurological or other medical symptoms but medical investigations are negative. As it turned out, this particular patient was well known to the staff as a patient with many emergency room visits and had been diagnosed with conversion disorder. That was the reason behind their calm. *Cautionary note:* Do not diagnose conversion disorder before doing the necessary investigation that rules out a medical condition. Moreover, these patients and their family and/or friends do need reassurance and education to help them deal with this illness.

Pain disorder

The main feature of this disorder is persistent, severe and distressing pain in one or more anatomical sites, which cannot be explained by any medical condition but, due to its severity, may warrant clinical attention. It affects the individual's daily functioning and the symptoms often occur in association with an emotional conflict or a psychological problem. These symptoms can result in increased attention from the family, friends and medical professionals. The level of impairment in functioning can be severe enough to preclude the ability to work or go to school, and result in overuse of medications. The pain becomes the focus of the individual's life, and may lead to disruptions in family and other relationships.

The DSM-IV mentions three subcategories of this disorder:

➥ *pain disorder associated with psychological factors:* psychological problems are found to be the main factor behind the onset and the maintenance of the pain disorder
➥ *pain disorder associated with both psychological factors and a general medical condition:* both conditions are found to be behind the onset of the disorder and play a role in exacerbations
➥ *pain disorder associated with a general medical condition:* a medical condition is the sole cause of the pain disorder without the presence of any contributing psychological problems. This subtype is generally listed under axis III of the multiaxial diagnosis in DSM-IV as a medical condition and not as a mental disorder.

Hypochondriasis

The essential feature of this disorder is a persistent preoccupation with the possibility of having one or more serious diseases due to the misinterpretation of one or more bodily signs or symptoms. The concern is not justified by any medical findings, and the person is not relieved by the physician's reassurance. The preoccupation affects one's social and occupational functioning and becomes the focus of one's life. The preoccupation may be with bodily functions (heartbeat, sweating . . .), minor physical abnormalities, vague, ambiguous sensations (aching veins, burning head . . .). Often, medical examinations and tests are sought. Despite negative results, patients will persist in their quest for a "diagnosis". Concern about the feared illness often becomes a focus of the person's self-image and a cause for family and relational problems.

Body dysmorphic disorder

The essential feature of body dysmorphic disorder is a preoccupation with a defect in one's appearance, which is either imagined or, if a slight abnormality is present, then the individual's concern is excessive and causes distress that is judged to be disproportionate. Complaints usually revolve around flaws in the face or head (acne, thinning hair, facial asymmetry, shape or size of eyes, nose, mouth . . .), or other body parts (breasts, arms, feet, buttocks . . .) or overall body size. There can be multiple preoccupations about different body parts at the same time. Individuals usually feel very ashamed and tormented by their "deformity" and find this worrying very hard to control. They may spend hours thinking about it, to the point that these thoughts dominate their lives and interfere with their daily functioning. Feelings of self-consciousness may lead them to avoid work, school and social situations.

Gender issues

The literature on anxiety and somatoform disorders in the Arab world reveals marked gender differences across several measures of these two constructs, with women in general having higher rates than men – which is also true of Western studies. Different authors have attempted to explain these findings in various ways, ranging from genetic and hormonal differences to social stereotyping.

One study distributed the Kuwait University Anxiety Scale (KUAS) to undergraduate students in 16 countries. In 11 out of the 16 countries – namely, Egypt, Iraq, Morocco, Kuwait, Oman, Qatar, Lebanon, Pakistan, Algiers, Yemen and Syria – females had significantly higher mean anxiety scores than did their male counterparts. The author hypothesizes that the sex-role stereotyping of women as helpless and dependent causes them to experience more worry, and to avoid a wider range of situations. Moreover, some women lack the opportunity to express themselves, and they tend to conceal their worries and anxieties, generating even higher levels of anxiety. Furthermore, there is a growing internal conflict in many women between their traditional role of getting married and raising children on the one hand, and having an education and working outside the home on the other. No significant gender differences in anxiety were found among participants from Saudi Arabia, Jordan, Sudan, the Emirates and Palestine. The author speculates that one reason why these countries revealed no such differences might be due to the distribution of economic and social statuses more equally among the genders in these countries.[30] However, this explanation does not seem plausible, given the preponderance of evidence to the contrary in the literature.[27,31-43] Rather, it is more likely that sampling issues may have affected the results in these countries.

Some authors have tried to explain contradictory reports of the low incidence of mental illness in Arab women. In their book entitled *Psychotherapy with the Arab Patient*, Chaleby and Racy (1999) mention that the under-representation of females in mental hospital data is due to the active attempt by the family to hide the illness in order not to hinder affected women's marriageability. Since cultural expectations in some Arab countries do not recognize any role for women except in marriage and procreation, unmarried or childless women may develop somatic symptoms that elicit sympathy from their surroundings and can even sometimes create an alibi of being too "physically ill" to marry and procreate.[13]

Conclusion

This chapter sought to highlight the main issues related to anxiety disorders and somatoform disorders as cited in the DSM-IV and ICD-10 in terms of diagnosis and characteristics, emphasizing the clinical presentations of these disorders in the Arab world. It is important for clinicians offering services to Arab populations to take into consideration the multifaceted nature of these problems, and, in particular, to consider the role of the family and community in providing support and assisting individuals in their recovery. This will help service providers in the consideration of an accurate diagnosis, and consequently, suitable treatment for patients. Future research is needed to explore culturally relevant features of anxiety disorders, precipitating and protective factors, and the role of the family in detection, treatment and outcomes.

References

1 El-Islam MF. Cultural aspects of illness behavior. *Arab Journal of Psychiatry* 1995; **6 (1):** 13–18.

2 World Health Organization. *The ICD-10 Classification of Mental and Behavioural Disorders: clinical descriptions and diagnostic guidelines.* Geneva: World Health Organization; 1992.

3 American Psychiatric Association. Task Force on DSM-IV. *Diagnostic and Statistical Manual of Mental Disorders: DSM-IV.* 4th ed. Washington, DC: American Psychiatric Association; 1994.

4 Karam EG, Mneimneh ZN, Karam AN *et al.* Prevalence and treatment of mental disorders in Lebanon: a national epidemiological survey. *Lancet* 2006; **367 (9515):** 1000–6.

5 Okasha A, Kamel M, Sadek A *et al.* Psychiatric morbidity among university students in Egypt. *Br J Psychiatry* 1977; **131:** 149–54.

6 Okasha A, Ashour A. Psycho-demographic study of anxiety in Egypt: the PSE in its Arabic version. *Br J Psychiatry* 1981; **139:** 70–3.

7 Kessler RC, Davis CG, Kendler KS. Childhood adversity and adult psychiatric disorder in the US National Comorbidity Survey. *Psychol Med* 1997; **27 (5):** 1101–19.

8 Abdel-Khalek AM. Death anxiety in Spain and five Arab countries. *Psychol Rep* 2003; **93 (2):** 527–8.

 9 Abdel-Khalek AM, Lester D. Anxiety in Kuwaiti and American college students. *Psychol Rep* 2006; **99 (2):** 512–14.

10 Eapen V, Ghubash R, Salem MO *et al.* Familial predictors of childhood shyness: a study of the United Arab Emirates population. *Community Genet* 2005; **8 (1):** 61–4.

11 Chaleby K. Social phobia in Saudis. *Soc Psychiatry* 1987; **22 (3):** 167–70.

12 Chaleby KS, Raslan A. Delineation of social phobia in Saudia Arabians. *Soc Psychiatry Psychiatr Epidemiol* 1990; **25 (6):** 324–7.

13 El-Islam MF. Cultural aspects of morbid fears in Qatari women. *Soc Psychiatry Psychiatr Epidemiol* 1994; **29 (3):** 137–40.

14 Weissman MM, Bland RC, Canino GJ *et al.* The cross-national epidemiology of panic disorder. *Arch Gen Psychiatry* 1997; **54 (4):** 305–9.

15 Al-Issa I. Religion and psychopathology. In: Al-Issa I, editor. *Al-Junun: mental illness in the Islamic world.* Madison, CT: International Universities Press Inc.; 2000. pp. 14–15.

16 Al-Issa I, Oudji S. Culture and anxiety disorders. In: Kazarian SS, Evans R, editors. *Cultural Clinical Psychology: theory, research and practice.* New York: Oxford University Press; 1998. pp. 127–51.

17 Karam E. Psychosocial consequences of war among civilian populations. *Current Opinion in Psychiatry* 2003; **16 (4):** 413–19.

18 Punamaki RL, Komproe IH, Qouta S *et al.* The role of peritraumatic dissociation and gender in the association between trauma and mental health in a Palestinian community sample. *Am J Psychiatry* 2005; **162 (3):** 545–51.

19 Farhood L, Noureddine SN. PTSD, depression and health status in Lebanese civilians exposed to a church explosion. *International Journal of Psychiatry in Medicine* 2003; **33 (1):** 39–53.

20 Thabet AA, Vostanis P. Post-traumatic stress reactions in children of war. *J Child Psychol Psychiatry* 1999; **40 (3):** 385–91.

21 Van der Kolk BA, Pelcovitz D, Roth S *et al.* Dissociation, somatization, and affect dysregulation: the complexity of adaptation of trauma. *Am J Psychiatry* 1996; **153 (7 Suppl):** 83–93.

22 Naja WJ, Pelissolo A, Haddad RS *et al.* A general population survey on patterns of benzodiazepine use and dependence in Lebanon. *Acta Psychiatr Scand* 2000; **102 (6):** 429–31.

23 Karam EG, Yabroudi PF, Melhem NM. Comorbidity of substance abuse and other psychiatric disorders in acute general psychiatric admissions: a study from Lebanon. *Compr Psychiatry* 2002; **43 (6):** 463–8.

24 Okasha A. Focus on psychiatry in Egypt. *Br J Psychiatry* 2004; **185:** 266–72.

25 El-Rufaie OE, Al-Sabosy MA, Bener A *et al.* Somatized mental disorder among primary care Arab patients. I. Prevalence and clinical and sociodemographic characteristics. *J Psychosom Res* 1999; **46 (6):** 549–55.

26 Sayed M. Conceptualization of mental illness within Arab cultures: meeting challenges in cross-cultural settings. *Social Behavior and Personality* 2003; **31 (4):** 333–42.

27 Al-Habeeb T, Abdulgani Y, Al-Ghamdi M *et al.* The sociodemographic and clinical pattern of hysteria in Saudi Arabia. *Arab Journal of Psychiatry* 1999; **10 (2).**

28 Shunaigat W. Clinical characteristics of conversion disorder in Jordan. *Arab Journal of Psychiatry* 2001; **12 (1):** 38–44.

29 Bener A, Saad AG, Micallef R *et al.* Sociodemographic and clinical characteristics of patients with dissociative disorders in an Arabian society. *Med Princ Pract* 2006; **15 (5):** 362–7.

30 Alansari B. Gender differences in anxiety among undergraduates from sixteen Islamic countries. *Social Behavior and Personality* 2006; **34 (6):** 651–60.

31 Dwairy M. Parenting styles and mental health of Palestinian-Arab adolescents in Israel. *Transcult Psychiatry* 2004; **41 (2):** 233–52.

32 Abou Shabana K, el-Shiek M, el-Nazer M *et al.* Women's perceptions and practices regarding their rights to reproductive health. *East Mediterr Health J* 2003; **9 (3):** 296–308.

33 Abou-Saleh MT, Ghubash R, Daradkeh TK. Al Ain Community Psychiatric Survey. I. Prevalence and socio-demographic correlates. *Soc Psychiatry Psychiatr Epidemiol* 2001; **36 (1):** 20–8.

34 Al Ma'aitah R, Haddad L, Umlauf MG. Health promotion behaviors of Jordanian women. *Health Care Women Int* 1999; **20 (6):** 533–46.

35 Al-Hosani HA, Brebner J, Bener AB *et al.* Study of mortality risk factors for children under age 5 in Abu Dhabi. *East Mediterr Health J* 2003; **9 (3):** 333–43.

36 Al-Krenawi A, Graham J, Izzeldin A. The psychosocial impact of polygamous marriages on Palestinian women. *Women and Health* 2001; **34 (1):** 1–16.

37 Al-Krenawi A, Graham JR. Gender and biomedical/traditional mental health utilization among the Bedouin-Arabs of the Negev. *Cult Med Psychiatry* 1999; **23 (2):** 219–43.

38 Al-Krenawi A, Graham JR, Kandah J. Gendered utilization differences of mental health services in Jordan. *Community Ment Health J* 2000; **36 (5):** 501–11.

39 Al-Krenawi A, Wiesel-Lev R. Attitudes toward and perceived psychosocial impact of female circumcision as practiced among the Bedouin-Arabs of the Negev. *Fam Process* 1999; **38 (4):** 431–43.

40 Al-Sawaf M, Al-Issa I. Sex and sexual dysfunction in an Arab-Islamic society. In: Al-Issa I, editor. *Al-Junun: mental illness in the Islamic world.* Madison, CT: International Universities Press Inc.; 2000. pp. 295–311.

41 Daradkeh T, Alawan A, Al-Ma'aitah R *et al.* Psychiatric morbidity and its sociodemographic correlates among women in Irbid, Jordan. *East Mediterr Health J* 2006; **12 (Suppl 2):** S-107–S-117.

42 De Jong J, Shepherd B, Mortagy I *et al. The Reproductive Health of Young People in the Middle East and North Africa.* Tours; 2005.

43 Fargues P. Women in Arab countries: challenging the patriarchal system? *Reprod Health Matters* 2005; **13 (25):** 43–8.

CHAPTER 13

Post-traumatic stress disorder

⟨* Eyad El-Sarraj, Taysir Diab and Abdel Aziz Thabet

Introduction

Post-traumatic stress disorder (PTSD) develops after a person sees, is involved in or hears of an extreme, sudden, unexpected and unavoidable traumatic stressor. The person reacts to this experience with intense fear, horror or help-lessness, persistently relives the event, and tries to avoid being reminded of it. To make the diagnosis, the symptoms must last for more than a month after the event and must significantly affect important areas of daily life such as family and work.

The text revision of the *Diagnostic and Statistical Manual of Mental Disorders* 4th edition (DSM-IV-TR) defines a disorder that is similar to PTSD, has been termed "acute stress disorder" (ASD) and is categorized by the *International Classification of Diseases* (ICD-10) as "acute stress reaction". This response occurs earlier than PTSD (within four weeks of the event) and remits within between two days to four weeks. If symptoms persist after this time, a diagnosis of PTSD is warranted.

The events causing both ASD and PTSD are overwhelming enough to affect almost anyone. They can arise from natural catastrophes or human-induced events like war, imprisonment, torture, assault, rape and serious accidents. Persons re-experience the traumatic event as intrusive thoughts and images in their dreams and daily thoughts. These thoughts and images are accompanied by marked anxiety and other states of hyperarousal. To compensate for this, the sufferers try to avoid anything that would bring the event to mind ("triggers"), and they undergo a numbing of responsiveness resulting in detachment from their emotions and from others. Other associated symptoms include depression and cognitive difficulties such as poor concentration.

History

"Soldier's heart" or "irritable heart" was the term applied to soldiers who suffered from a syndrome similar to PTSD during the US Civil War. In the 1900s psychoanalysts, particularly in the United States, applied the diagnosis of "traumatic neurosis" to the condition. In World War I, the syndrome was called "shell shock". In World War II, veterans, and survivors of the atomic bombings in Japan with similar symptoms, were labeled as suffering from "combat neurosis or operational fatigue". The psychiatric morbidity associated with Vietnam War veterans resulted in the concept of "post-traumatic stress disorder", as it is currently termed.

Epidemiology

The prevalence of PTSD varies according to the exposure to traumatic events of the population studied. General population rates in the West are around 1–3%. Among high-risk groups whose members experienced traumatic events, the lifetime prevalence rates range from 5% to 75%. Reported rates among crime victims are between 19% and 75%, and rates as high as 80% have been reported following rape. In Gaza, a city in Palestinian Authority area, one study conducted by the Gaza Community Mental Health Program (GCMHP) in 1996 reported that prevalence rates of PTSD among ex-political prisoners were 30%.[1]

Although PTSD can appear at any age, it is most prevalent in young adults, because they tend be more exposed to precipitating situations. Children can also have the disorder. Men and women differ in the types of traumas to which they are exposed and their liability to develop PTSD.[2] The lifetime prevalence is significantly higher in women, and higher proportions of women go on to develop the disorder.[3] The disorder is most likely to occur in those who are single, divorced, widowed, socially withdrawn or of low socioeconomic status. The most important risk factors for the disorder, however, are the severity, duration and proximity of a person's exposure to the actual trauma. First-degree biological relatives of persons with a history of depression have an increased risk for developing PTSD following a traumatic event, suggesting that there may be a biological predisposition to the disorder.

Co-morbidity

Co-morbidity rates are high among patients with PTSD; about two-thirds suffer from at least two other psychiatric disorders. Common co-morbid conditions include mood disorders (depressive or bipolar disorders), substance-related disorders and other anxiety disorders, sometimes with psychotic manifestations. Co-morbid disorders increase the predisposition to PTSD and vice-versa.

Etiology

The subjective meaning of the trauma to the individual is another important factor that can influence the development or severity of PTSD. This is illustrated by the observation that, though a traumatic event is a necessary causative factor in the development of PTSD, not everyone experiences the disorder after exposure to the same event. Therefore, trauma alone does not suffice to cause the disorder. Other pre-existing biological, psychosocial factors and life events taking place before and/or after the trauma should also be considered.

Studies have found that risk factors for the development of PTSD include: a history of childhood trauma; the presence of borderline, paranoid, dependent or antisocial personality traits; inadequate family or peer support; being female; genetic vulnerability to psychiatric illness; recent stressful life changes; a recent medical illness; and recent excessive substance or alcohol intake.

Complex psychodynamic, cognitive-behavioral and neurochemical models of PTSD have been proposed.[4]

The psychodynamic model

This model hypothesizes that the trauma has reactivated a previously quiescent, yet unresolved psychological conflict. The revival of the childhood trauma results in regression and the use of the defense mechanisms of repression, denial, reaction formation and undoing. According to Freud, a "splitting of consciousness" occurs in patients who reported a history of childhood sexual trauma. A pre-existing conflict might symbolically be reawakened by a new traumatic event.

The cognitive-behavioral model

This model posits that individuals affected by PTSD are unable to fully process or rationalize the trauma that precipitated the disorder. The brain intermittently continues to attempt to process the information, triggering attempts to evade it through cognitions and behaviors aimed at interfering with re-experiencing the trauma.[5] Consistent with their partial ability to cope cognitively with the event, persons experience alternating periods of acknowledging and blocking the event.

The behavioral aspect of PTSD emphasizes two phases in its development. First, the trauma (the unconditioned stimulus) that produces a fear response is paired, through classical conditioning, with a conditioned stimulus (physical or mental reminders of the trauma, such as sights, smells or sounds). Second, through instrumental learning, the conditioned stimuli elicit the fear response independent of the original unconditioned stimulus, and persons develop a pattern of avoiding both the conditioned and the unconditioned stimuli. Some persons may also inadvertently receive secondary gain due to the condition, including monetary compensation, increased attention and the fulfillment of dependency needs. This reinforces the disorder and leads to its persistence.

The neuro-chemical model

Basic studies of animal responses to stress have led to neurochemical and neuro-physical theories involving norepinephrine, dopamine, endogenous opioids and benzodiazepine receptors and the hypothalamic-pituitary-adrenal (HPA) axis.[6]

Measures of biological variables in clinical populations have supported the hypotheses that the noradrenergic and endogenous opioid systems, as well as the HPA axis, are hyperactive in some individuals with PTSD. Other biological findings include increased activity and responsiveness of the autonomic nervous system, as evidenced by elevated heart rates and blood pressure readings and by abnormal sleep patterns (e.g. increased rapid eye movement (REM) sleep and decreased REM-latency).

Animal studies have shown that stress is associated with structural changes in the hippocampus, and studies of combat veterans with PTSD have revealed lower average volumes in the hippocampal region of the brain compared with matched controls.[7] Furthermore, researchers suggest that the hippocampus is not necessarily the only area of the brain to show structural changes in PTSD; studies of depression have shown similar changes in the amygdala and prefrontal cortex.

Diagnosis

The DSM-IV-TR diagnostic criteria for PTSD specify that the symptoms of experiencing, avoidance and hyperarousal must have lasted more than one month. For patients whose symptoms have been present less than one month, the appropriate diagnosis may be ASD (*see* Chapter 12, Anxiety and somatoform disorders).

DSM-IV-TR diagnostic criteria for PTSD allow clinicians to specify whether the disorder is acute (if the symptoms have lasted less than three months) or chronic (if the symptoms have lasted three months or longer). DSM-IV-TR also allows clinicians to specify that the disorder had a delayed onset if the commencement of the symptoms was six months or more after the stressful event.

Clinical features

The principal clinical features of PTSD are a painful re-experiencing of the event, a pattern of avoidance and emotional numbing, and fairly constant hyper-arousal. The disorder may not develop until months or even years after the event. The mental status examination often reveals feelings of guilt, rejection and humiliation. Patients may also describe dissociative states and panic attacks. Illusions and hallucinations may be present. Associated symptoms can include aggression, violence, poor impulse control, depression and substance-related disorders. Cognitive testing may reveal that patients have impaired memory and attention.

PTSD in children and adolescents

PTSD occurs in children and adolescents, but most studies of the disorder have focused on adults. The DSM-IV-TR has little to say about PTSD as it affects young children except to describe symptoms such as repetitive dreams of the event, nightmares of monsters, and the development of physical symptoms such as stomachaches and headaches.

High rates of PTSD have been documented in children exposed to such life-threatening events as combat and other war-related trauma, kidnapping, severe illness or burns, bone marrow transplantation, and a number of natural or human-induced disasters. As might be expected, the prevalence of PTSD is higher in children than in adults exposed to the same stressor. Circumstances in which children are exposed to nearly continuous violence, such as the current situation in many of the Palestinian Authority areas, result in up to 90% of children developing the disorder. One study conducted by the GCMHP showed that 32.4% of Palestinian children living under severe conditions during the last years of the Al-Aqsa Intifada developed acute PTSD symptoms, while 44.4% of them suffered from moderate levels of PTSD symptoms.

Child risk factors include demographic factors (e.g. age, sex, socioeconomic status), other life events (positive and negative), social and cultural cognitions, psychiatric co-morbidity, and inherent coping strategies. Family factors (e.g. parental psychopathology and function, material status and education) play key roles in determining child symptoms. Parents' response to traumatic events particularly influence young children who may not completely understand the nature of the trauma or its inherent danger.[8]

Precipitants of PTSD in children may be sudden, single-incident trauma or ongoing or chronic trauma such as physical or sexual abuse. Children may also suffer as the result of "indirect" exposure – that is, the unwitnessed death or injury of a loved one, as in situations of disaster, war or community violence.

Children, like adults, re-experience the traumatic event in the form of distressing, intrusive thoughts or memories, flashbacks and dreams. Children's nightmares may be linked specifically to a traumatic theme or may generalize to other fears. Flashbacks occur in children as well as in their adolescent or adult victim counterparts.

Traumatic play, a specific form of re-experiencing seen in young children, consists of repetitive acting-out of the trauma or trauma-related themes in play. Older children may incorporate aspects of the trauma into their lives in a process termed "re-enactment". Fantasized actions of intervention or revenge are common; adolescents with PTSD should be considered at increased risk for impulsive acting-out secondary to anger and revenge fantasies. Related behaviors in child and adolescent victims of trauma include sexual acting-out, substance use and delinquency. Children often withdraw and show reduced interest in previously enjoyable activities[9]. Habits like thumb-sucking, nail-biting and other regressive behaviors such as enuresis, mutism or fear of sleeping alone may also occur.

Differential diagnosis

A major consideration in the diagnosis of PTSD is the possibility that the patient also incurred a head injury during the trauma. Other organic considerations that can both cause and exacerbate the symptoms are epilepsy, and alcohol and other substance-related disorders. Clinicians must consider the diagnosis of PTSD in patients who have somatoform pain disorder, other anxiety disorders, borderline personality disorder, dissociative disorders, factitious disorders and malingering.

Course and prognosis

PTSD usually develops some time after the trauma. The onset can be as short as one week or as long as thirty years.[10] Symptoms can fluctuate over time and may be most intense during periods of stress. Untreated, about 30% of patients recover completely, 40% continue to have mild symptoms, 20% continue to have moderate symptoms, and 10% remain unchanged or become worse. After one year, about 50% of patients will recover. A good prognosis is predicted by rapid onset of the symptoms, short duration of the symptoms, good pre-morbid functioning, strong social supports, and the absence of other psychiatric, medical or substance-related disorders or other risk factors.

Cultural issues related to PTSD

Culture has been defined by sociologists and anthropologists in different ways. Most would agree that it refers to a number of collective factors. These include patterns of behavior and customs, values, beliefs and attitudes, implicit rules of conduct, patterns of family and social organization, and taboos and sanctions. These are shared by a group of people who have a common identity, based on ethnic and sometimes territorial unity.[11]

Family and social support is often difficult to distinguish from underlying cultural factors. Cultural differences are evident in the responses of people to traumatic events and the presentation of psychopathology. In a study of South Asian refugee children who settled in Australia, South Asian children showed higher rates of somatoform symptoms than did the general Australian child population.[12]

Similar physical presentations of distress have been found in other non-Western traumatized populations, such as Lebanese children, 58% of whom suffered from somatoform disorders four years after the Israeli invasion of Lebanon in 1982.[13] Farhood *et al.* also found high rates of somatization among Lebanese children and parents.[14]

Similarly, Palestinian children suffering from PTSD in the West Bank were found to suffer predominantly from conduct and psychosomatic problems. In addition, conduct and psychosomatic problems were more severe within the refugee camps than in urban or rural areas.[15] In another study of Palestinians living in Gaza exposed to traumatic events during the First Intifada, it was reported that 25% suffered from conversion fits.[16] This presentation applied to both children and adults.

The role of culture in an individual's experience of PTSD, as well as the function of culture in providing strategies to overcome the disorder, have been explored. Adolescent refugees from Cambodia who lived in the United States were likely to continue to feel guilty about abandoning their homeland, be haunted by painful memories, or have impaired concentration, compared to Cambodian adolescents in Australia where there was less pressure to conform, and where they were able to attend some traditional ceremonies.[17] The development of PTSD among Palestinian children seemed to be partially mediated by family and community attitudes and support.[18]

Unlike conditions such as schizophrenia or depression, the diagnostic category of PTSD is a relatively new one. Therefore, there are few studies that address cultural aspects of this disorder. However, it is clear that cultural factors have an important role to play in the genesis and presentation of PTSD and how it is perceived, responded to and treated.[18] It has been reported that individuals in Arab countries may preferentially express psychological problems through somatic symptoms like headaches, abdominal pains and conversion fits,[2,13,19,20] therefore, cultural factors must be taken into account in evaluation and treatment.

Management of PTSD

Despite the notable increase in the quantity and quality of empirical research in the area of trauma and PTSD in recent years, there have been few rigorous studies of treatment outcomes of populations with this disorder.

A variety of modalities have been presented in descriptive papers, including individual, family, group, behavior and self-inoculation therapy, as well as psychopharmacological treatment. Unfortunately, there has been limited evidence of the effectiveness of various treatment interventions, or the comparative advantages and specificity of therapeutic modalities. A recent study in the United States that evaluated women who were suffering from PTSD and randomized to receive "prolonged exposure therapy" (a type of cognitive behavioral therapy) or another type of supportive therapy, reported significantly greater benefits in both short- and long-term outcomes with the patients receiving prolonged exposure therapy.[21]

Traditionally, major approaches for clients with acute PTSD have included support, encouragement to discuss the event, and education in a variety of coping mechanisms (e.g. relaxation). When an individual has delayed-onset PTSD, the emphasis should be on education about the disorder and its treatment.

Drug therapy

Anti-depressant drugs – selective serotonin re-uptake inhibitors (SSRIs) such as sertraline (Zoloft) or paroxetine (Paxil) – are considered first-line treatments for PTSD owing to their efficacy, tolerability and safety. Other medications such as imipramine (Tofranil) and amitriptyline (Elatrol), two tricyclic drugs, may also be used in the treatment of PTSD. Dosages of imipramine and amitriptyline should be the same as those used to treat depressive disorders, and an adequate trial should last at least six to eight weeks. Patients who respond well should prob-ably continue the pharmacotherapy for at least one year before an attempt is made to withdraw the medication. Some studies indicate that pharmacotherapy is more effective in treating the depression, anxiety and hyperarousal than in treating the avoidance, denial and emotional numbing.[22] Other drugs that may be useful in the treatment of PTSD include buspirone (BuSpar) and trazodone (Desyrel), which are predominantly serotonergic in action, monoamine oxidase inhibitors such as phenelzine (Nardil), and some anticonvulsants such as car-bamazipine (Tegretol) or valproate (Depakene). Use of clonidine (Catapres) and propranolol (Inderal), which are anti-adrenergic agents, might theoreti-cally be effective given the noradrenergic hyperactivity in the disorder. There is little evidence that antipsychotic drugs are effective in this disorder. Therefore the use of medications such as haloperidol (Haldol) should be reserved for the short-term control of severe aggression and agitation.

Although anxiolytics such as benzodiazepines would be expected to be very effective in this condition, at least one study has shown only modest improve-ment in associated anxiety, and no significant change in the underlying PTSD symptoms.[23] Given the strong association between PTSD and substance abuse, careful consideration should be given to the risks and benefits of these agents prior to considering their use in individuals with PTSD.

Psychotherapy

Psychotherapy may be useful in the treatment of many patients with PTSD. Psychotherapeutic interventions for PTSD include behavioral therapy, cognitive therapy and hypnosis. Many clinicians advocate time-limited psychotherapy for the victims of trauma. This therapy usually takes a cognitive approach and also provides support and security. The short-term nature of the psychotherapy minimizes the risk of dependence and chronicity, but issues of suspicion, paranoia and trust may adversely affect compliance. Therapists should overcome patients' denial of the traumatic event, encourage them to relax, and remove them from the source of the stress. Patients should be encouraged to sleep, using medication if necessary. Support from persons in their environment (such as friends and relatives) should be provided. Patients should be encouraged to review and abreact emotional feelings associated with the traumatic event, and to plan for future recovery. Abreaction (releasing or experiencing the emotions associated with the event) may be helpful for some patients.

Psychotherapy after a traumatic event should follow a model of crisis intervention with support, education and the development of coping mechanisms and acceptance of the event. In some cases, reconstruction of the traumatic events with associated abreaction and catharsis may be helpful.

Therapeutic considerations in traumatized children

Pynoos and Nader described a "psychological first-aid" approach for children exposed to community violence, which may be offered in schools as well as in traditional treatment settings. This model is based on clarifying the traumatic event, normalizing children's PTSD reactions, encouraging the expression of feelings, teaching problem-solving techniques, and referring the most symptomatic children for ongoing specialist treatment.[24] Individual therapy begins with a sensitive clinical interview. The desire to avoid reminders of the trauma commonly dampens the child's verbal expression. Some authors maintain that play therapy is beneficial for children with PTSD.[25]

Galante and Foa (1986) evaluated a school-based group therapy for high-risk Italian children victims of a devastating earthquake. Children were evaluated at six and 18 months post-earthquake. The children who had received the treatment showed a significant drop in PTSD symptoms.[26]

Group therapy and support groups have been used in children exposed to traumatic events on a large scale. Studies found that group therapy was ideal in educating youths and adults about their symptoms and in providing age-appropriate explanations. In studies of Southeast Asian refugees who had suffered the death of a parent, children in group psychotherapy had better outcomes than did the control group.[27,28]

Another advantage of groups for traumatized children may include their cost-effectiveness over individual treatment.

Practitioners should note, however, there may also be disadvantages in group work. Not all children feel comfortable sharing in a group, and some need more intensive individual treatment. Group discussion has the potential to re-traumatize children through re-exposure to their own experiences or those of others (children may prematurely adopt other young people's coping strategies before fully examining their own responses). It is important to set limits on the expression of anger and aggression, which may create anxiety in peers and which may require individual work.[29]

Chemtob, Nakashima and Carlson found that three group therapy sessions resulted in substantial reduction of PTSD, anxiety and depressive symptoms in children with prolonged psychopathology, following exposure to a hurricane in Hawaii one year earlier, compared with waiting list controls.[30] There has been even more limited evidence regarding the application of such programs in children who experienced war trauma.[31]

One study evaluated the short-term impact of a *group crisis intervention* for children aged from nine to 15 years from five refugee camps in the Gaza strip during the ongoing military conflict. Children were allocated to group intervention encouraging expression of experiences and emotions through storytelling, drawing, free play and role-play; education about symptoms; or no intervention. No significant impact of the group intervention was established on children's post-traumatic or depressive symptoms. It is possible that the passive nature of the intervention, or continuing ongoing exposure to trauma, affected the outcome.[32]

Field *et al.* (1996) evaluated the impact of *massage therapy* or a video attention-control condition in children exposed to Hurricane Andrew. The massage therapy group experienced significantly more improvement in PTSD symptoms than did the control group. This study thus supported the use of muscle relaxation techniques in children with PTSD,[33] however, such interventions usually target small numbers of children and may not be cost-effective. They may also be less acceptable to parents in this society.

Deblinger *et al.* used trauma-focused *cognitive-behavioral therapy* (CBT) to treat sexually abused children by one of four treatment conditions: child-only receiving CBT, parent-only receiving CBT, child and parent receiving CBT, or assignment to a community treatment control. Results indicated that, although symptoms improved in all groups, the two conditions in which the child received direct treatment demonstrated significantly greater improvement in PTSD symptoms than did the other two interventions.[34]

Goenjian and colleagues (1997) found that youths who received *brief trauma/ grief-focused psychotherapy* after an earthquake in Armenia had significantly fewer PTSD symptoms in all three symptom clusters, while the severity of these symptoms increased significantly among the subjects not treated.[35] In an intervention study of sexually abused children, the experimental group that received brief focused individual psychotherapy exhibited significantly greater improvement after one year than did children who had received non-directive supportive therapy.[36]

Cognitive-behavioral interventions, mainly in group settings, have been associated with observed decreases in PTSD symptoms among children who experienced single-incident stressors[37] and sexual abuse.[38]

References

1 El Sarraj E, Punamaki RL, Salmi S *et al.* Experiences of torture and ill-treatment and posttraumatic stress disorder symptoms among Palestinian political prisoners. *J Trauma Stress* 1996; **9 (3):** 595–606.

2 Punamaki RL, Komproe IH, Qouta S *et al.* The role of peritraumatic dissociation and gender in the association between trauma and mental health in a Palestinian community sample. *Am J Psychiatry* 2005; **162 (3):** 545–51.

3 Tolin DF, Foa EB. Sex differences in trauma and posttraumatic stress disorder: a quantitative review of 25 years of research. *Psychol Bull* 2006; **132 (6):** 959–92.

4 Geracioti TD, Jr, Baker DG, Ekhator NN *et al.* CSF norepinephrine concentrations in posttraumatic stress disorder. *Am J Psychiatry* 2001; **158 (8):** 1227–30.

5 Meiser-Stedman R. Towards a cognitive-behavioral model of PTSD in children and adolescents. *Clin Child Fam Psychol Rev* 2002; **5 (4):** 217–32.

6 Miller MM, McEwen BS. Establishing an agenda for translational research on PTSD. *Ann N Y Acad Sci* 2006; **1071:** 294–312.

7 Bremner JD, Randall P, Scott TM *et al.* MRI-based measurement of hippocampal volume in patients with combat-related posttraumatic stress disorder. *Am J Psychiatry* 1995; **152 (7):** 973–81.

8 Qouta S, Punamaki RL, El Sarraj E. Prevalence and determinants of PTSD among Palestinian children exposed to military violence. *Eur Child Adolesc Psychiatry* 2003; **12 (6):** 265–72.

9 Thabet AA, Abed Y, Vostanis P. Comorbidity of PTSD and depression among refugee children during war conflict. *J Child Psychol Psychiatry* 2004; **45 (3):** 533–42.

10 Carty J, O'Donnell ML, Creamer M. Delayed-onset PTSD: a prospective study of injury survivors. *J Affect Disord* 2006; **90 (2–3):** 257–61.

11 De Silva P. Cultural aspects of post traumatic stress disorder. In: Yule W, editor. *Post Traumatic Stress Disorder: concept and therapy.* Chichester: John Wiley and Sons; 1999. pp. 116–17.

12 Krupinski J, Burrows GD. *The Price of Freedom: young Indochinese refugees in Australia.* Sydney, New York: Pergamon Press; 1986.

13 Ryhida J, Shaya M, Armenian H. Child health in a city at war. In: Bryce JW, Armenian HK, editors. *In Wartime: the state of children in Lebanon.* Beirut, Lebanon: Jamiyah al-Kuwaytiyah li-Taqaddum al-Tufulah al-Arabiyah, Arab Gulf Programme for United Nations Development Organizations, American University of Beirut; 1986. p. xviii, 202.

14 Farhood L, Zurayk H, Chaya M *et al.* The impact of war on the physical and mental health of the family: the Lebanese experience. *Soc Sci Med* 1993; **36 (12):** 1555–67.

15 Baker AM. The psychological impact of the Intifada on Palestinian children in the occupied West Bank and Gaza: an exploratory study. *Am J Orthopsychiatry* 1990; **60 (4):** 496–505.

16 Hein FA, Qouta S, Thabet A *et al.* Trauma and mental health of children in Gaza. *BMJ* 1993; **306 (6885):** 1130–1.

17 Eisenbruch M. From post-traumatic stress disorder to cultural bereavement: diagnosis of Southeast Asian refugees. *Soc Sci Med* 1991; **33 (6):** 673–80.

18 Baker A, Shalhoub-Kevorkian N. Effects of political and military traumas on children: the Palestinian case. *Clin Psychol Rev* 1999; **19 (8):** 935–50.

19 Kirmayer LJ. Cultural variations in the clinical presentation of depression and anxiety: implications for diagnosis and treatment. *J Clin Psychiatry* 2001; **62 Suppl 13:** 22–8; discussion 29–30.

20 Becker SM. Detection of somatization and depression in primary care in Saudi Arabia. *Soc Psychiatry Psychiatr Epidemiol* 2004; **39 (12):** 962–6.

21 Schnurr PP, Friedman MJ, Engel CC *et al.* Cognitive behavioral therapy for posttraumatic stress disorder in women: a randomized controlled trial. *JAMA* 2007; **297 (8):** 820–30.

22 Marshall RD, Beebe KL, Oldham M *et al.* Efficacy and safety of paroxetine treatment for chronic PTSD: a fixed-dose, placebo-controlled study. *Am J Psychiatry* 2001; **158 (12):** 1982–8.

23 Braun P, Greenberg D, Dasberg H *et al.* Core symptoms of posttraumatic stress disorder unimproved by alprazolam treatment. *J Clin Psychiatry* 1990; **51 (6):** 236–8.

24 Pynoos R, Nader K. Psychological first aid and treatment approach to children exposed to community violence: research implications. *J Trauma Stress* 1988; **1:** 444–73.

25 Terr LC. Psychic trauma in children and adolescents. *Psychiatr Clin North Am* 1985; **8 (4):** 815–35.

26 Galante R, Foa D. An epidemiological study of psychic trauma and treatment effectivenesss for children after a natural disaster. *J Am Acad Child Psychiatry* 1986; **25:** 357–63.

27 Kinzie JD, Leung P, Bui A *et al.* Group therapy with Southeast Asian refugees. *Community Ment Health J* 1988; **24 (2):** 157–66.

28 Yule W, Williams R. Post traumatic stress reactions in children. *J Trauma Stress* 1990; **3:** 279–95.

29 Gillis H. Individual and small group psychotherapy for children involved in trauma and disaster. In: Saylor CF, editor. *Children and Disasters.* New York: Plenum Press; 1993. pp. 165–86.

30 Chemtob CM, Nakashima J, Carlson JG. Brief treatment for elementary school children with disaster-related posttraumatic stress disorder: a field study. *J Clin Psychol* 2002; **58 (1):** 99–112.

31 Ehntholt KA, Yule W. Practitioner review: assessment and treatment of refugee children and adolescents who have experienced war-related trauma. *J Child Psychol Psychiatry* 2006; **47 (12):** 1197–210.

32 Thabet AA, Vostanis P, Karim K. Group crisis intervention for children during ongoing war conflict. *Eur Child Adolesc Psychiatry* 2005; **14 (5):** 262–9.

33 Field T, Seligman S, Scafidi F *et al.* Alleviating posttraumatic stress in children following Hurricane Andrew. *J Appl Dev Psychol* 1996; **17:** 37–50.

34 Deblinger E, McLeer SV, Atkins MS *et al.* Post-traumatic stress in sexually abused, physically abused, and nonabused children. *Child Abuse Negl* 1989; **13 (3):** 403–8.

35 Goenjian AK, Karayan I, Pynoos RS *et al.* Outcome of psychotherapy among early adolescents after trauma. *Am J Psychiatry* 1997; **154 (4):** 536–42.

36 Cohen J, Mannarino A. A treatment outcome study for sexually abused preschool children: initial findings. *J Am Acad Child Adolesc Psychiatry* 1996; **35:** 42–50.

37 March JS, Amaya-Jackson L, Murray MC *et al.* Cognitive-behavioral psychotherapy for children and adolescents with posttraumatic stress disorder after a single-incident stressor. *J Am Acad Child Adolesc Psychiatry* 1998; **37 (6):** 585–93.

38 Cohen JA, Deblinger E, Mannarino AP *et al.* A multisite, randomized controlled trial for children with sexual abuse-related PTSD symptoms. *J Am Acad Child Adolesc Psychiatry* 2004; **43 (4):** 393–402.

CHAPTER 14

Eating disorders

(* *Nasser Shuriquie*

Introduction

Eating disorders have been classically perceived as Western culture-bound syndromes associated with culture-driven factors, such as unrealistic expectations of slenderness and attractiveness. These pressures are thought to have resulted from cultural changes in social standards, attitudes towards obesity, and the role of women. According to this hypothesis, the Western woman is under tremendous pressure from the media and peers to be slim and able to compete in a world controlled by men.

However, the drive to be thin is not universal, as cross-cultural studies have suggested.[1] It has been argued that in countries where food is scarce, plumpness is considered a feminine ideal.[2] Traditionally in Arab countries, plumpness has been considered attractive and a sign of womanhood and fertility.[3,4] This has led to the assumption that eating disorders are rare in Arab culture. Yet emerging evidence indicates that eating disorders are not uncommon in Arab countries, and that the numbers of individuals with abnormal eating attitudes and eating disorders may approximate international rates.[5-10] One hypothesis for the apparent emergence of these illnesses, which heretofore were thought to be non-existent in Arab countries, is that Arab women are experiencing conflicts between Western and Arab values through increased media exposure, travel and communication.[11]

Classification of eating disorders

What are the eating disorders? According to the *Diagnostic and Statistical Manual of Mental Disorders*, 4th edition (DSM-IV),[12] eating disorders are classified into:

- anorexia nervosa
- bulimia nervosa
- binge eating disorders
- eating disorders not otherwise specified
- feeding disorder of infancy and childhood.

The two main disorders, according to the *International Classification of Disease*, version 10 (ICD-10),[13] are anorexia nervosa and bulimia nervosa.

Anorexia nervosa

- Body weight is maintained at least 15% below expected weight or a BMI (kg/m^2) of 17.5 or less. Prepubertal patients may fail to gain weight during the period of growth.
- The weight loss is self-induced by specific avoidance of "fattening" foods, or by self-induced vomiting, purging, excessive exercise or the use of appetite suppressants or diuretics.
- Body image is distorted, such that there is persistent dread of fatness as an intrusive and overvalued idea. Also, the patient imposes a low weight threshold on himself/herself.
- An endocrine disorder that involves the hypothalamic/pituitary axis (HPA) may manifest in women as amenorrhea and in men as loss of sexual interest and potency.
- If the onset is prepubertal, it may result in delayed or arrested growth in children.

Bulimia nervosa

- There is a persistent preoccupation with eating and an irresistible craving for food.
- Individuals submit to episodes of massive overeating in short periods of time.
- The patient attempts to counteract weight gain by self-induced vomiting, and/or purgative abuse. The patient initiates periods of starvation or the use of appetite suppressants or diuretics.
- The psychopathology consists of a morbid dread of fatness, in which the patient sets herself a sharply defined weight threshold well below what would be a healthy optimum. There is often an earlier episode of anorexia nervosa.

Other eating disorders

Other disorders included in the ICD-10 are atypical anorexia nervosa, atypical bulimia nervosa, overeating and vomiting associated with other psychological disorders. The DSM-IV uses the term "eating disorder not otherwise specified" (EDNOS) for an eating disorder which does not quite meet the criteria for either anorexia nervosa or bulimia nervosa (atypical eating disorder).

Binge eating disorder

This disorder is not recognized in the ICD-10. It is classified as a research diagnostic criterion in the DSM-IV.

- There are recurrent episodes of binge eating.
- At least three of these symptoms are needed for the diagnosis: rapid eating; eating until discomfort occurs; eating without hunger; eating alone; self-disgust.
- The patient feels distress regarding binge eating.
- A frequency of episodes at least twice weekly for six months is required to make the diagnosis.
- The main difference from bulimia nervosa is the absence of inappropriate "compensatory behaviors", such as self-induced vomiting or using laxatives.

Eating disorders in Arab adolescent girls and women

Studies in Arab countries have found abnormal eating attitudes and excessive concerns about weight and shape among young females in Egypt,[8] Saudi Arabia,[6] Jordan,[9] the United Arab Emirates,[7] Oman,[5] and Qatar.[10] The Eating Attitude Test (EAT 40) devised by Garner and Garfinkel,[14] and translated and validated in Arab populations,[15] is a widely used screening instrument for eating attitudes.[16] One study reported that when the Arabic version of the EAT 40 was used to screen secondary school girls in Cairo, it was found that 11.4% of the girls had abnormal eating attitudes, and that 1.2% suffered from bulimia nervosa.[8] The author hypothesized that these adolescent girls were experiencing conflicts between Western values of autonomy and achievement, and traditional values of women as housewives and mothers. Al-Subaie and colleagues conducted a similar screening of female students in Saudi Arabia using the EAT 26 (a short version of the EAT 40) and found it useful and valid in screening large populations for eating disorders.[6] Both Nasser's and Al-Subaie's studies reported the EAT to be highly sensitive and reasonably specific in the Arab culture.

An exploratory study of 210 nursing students at two university colleges in Jordan using the Arabic version of the EAT 40 also indicated the presence of abnormal EAT (12.4%) and bulimia nervosa (0.99%) among the participants.[9] These figures are consistent with Western and other transcultural studies. On the other hand, an Omani study using the EAT reported that Omani teenagers (n=106) scored significantly higher than teenagers from other Western ethnic groups (n=87) and Omani adults (n=100). They found abnormal eating attitudes and behavior in 33% of the teenage sample. The study of the adult sample showed a 2% prevalence of anorexia nervosa, and a 1% prevalence of bulimia nervosa. The authors considered the emergence of eating disorders in Omani culture to be due to extensive economic and psychosocial changes in the region that conflict with traditional tribal and family values.[5]

A recent study conducted in United Arab Emirates on a representative random sample of 495 adolescent girls using the EAT 40 showed that 23.4% had abnormal eating attitudes and 2% had the full clinical syndrome of anorexia nervosa. The authors report that exposure to Western television programs was associated with the development of abnormal eating attitudes.[7]

These studies demonstrate that eating disorders are not restricted to Western societies. The world is increasingly becoming a global village through the influence of mass media; therefore Arab adolescents are exposed to the modern Western values of slimness and fitness as the most important aspects of beauty.

Shuriquie and Abdulhamid, using collective case study methodology, have examined the natural course and the outcome of eating disorders in five cases followed up for five years in Jordan.[17] An excerpt from their study provides a brief account of a five-year follow-up of a Jordanian woman with an eating disorder.

Case review: Miss "MS"

Miss MS is a 33-year-old, single architect, who lives in Amman with her family. She had a ten-year history of eating disorder prior her first presentation to us. The lowest weight she had ever reached was 35 kg. On presentation, she was clinically depressed and had suicidal thoughts and somatic complaints, felt isolated and had an extremely poor relationship with her family. She had been bingeing and purging on a regular basis (2–3 times daily). Her BMI was 16.54 on presentation and was diagnosed as a case of anorexia nervosa according to the ICD-10. She was engaged in motivation enhancement therapy (MET) – a form of interviewing aimed at improving an individual's intrinsic motivation to change. After treatment, she improved significantly, with reductions in the frequency of bingeing and self-induced vomiting.

The course of her illness was characterized by a fluctuating pattern, and was highly influenced by the strained relationship with her hostile family who had never been able to understand her illness. She went through a period of complete remission after the first six months of treatment, manifested by no abnormal weight control behaviors and improvement in social functioning. She established her own very successful architectural company. This improvement was probably related to her becoming increasingly motivated to change, as well as regular follow-ups, and taking fairly high doses of fluoxetine (a selective serotonin uptake inhibitor). This medication appeared to have reduced her urge to binge.

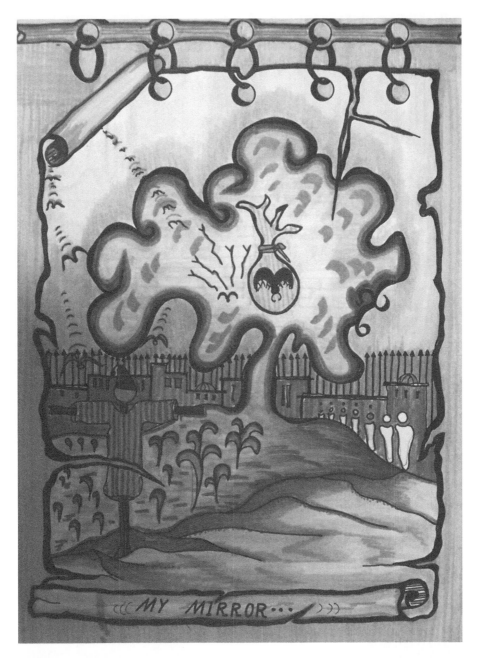

FIGURE 14.1 Miss MS drew a plastic bag of water hanging on a tree, which reflects the distorted and enlarged image of a bird. Such bags of water are used by farmers to scare birds away from fruit trees. She compares the way she sees herself in the mirror with the way birds see their deformed and enlarged reflection on the water bags. This drawing graphically illustrates the disturbance of body image in patients with eating disorders.

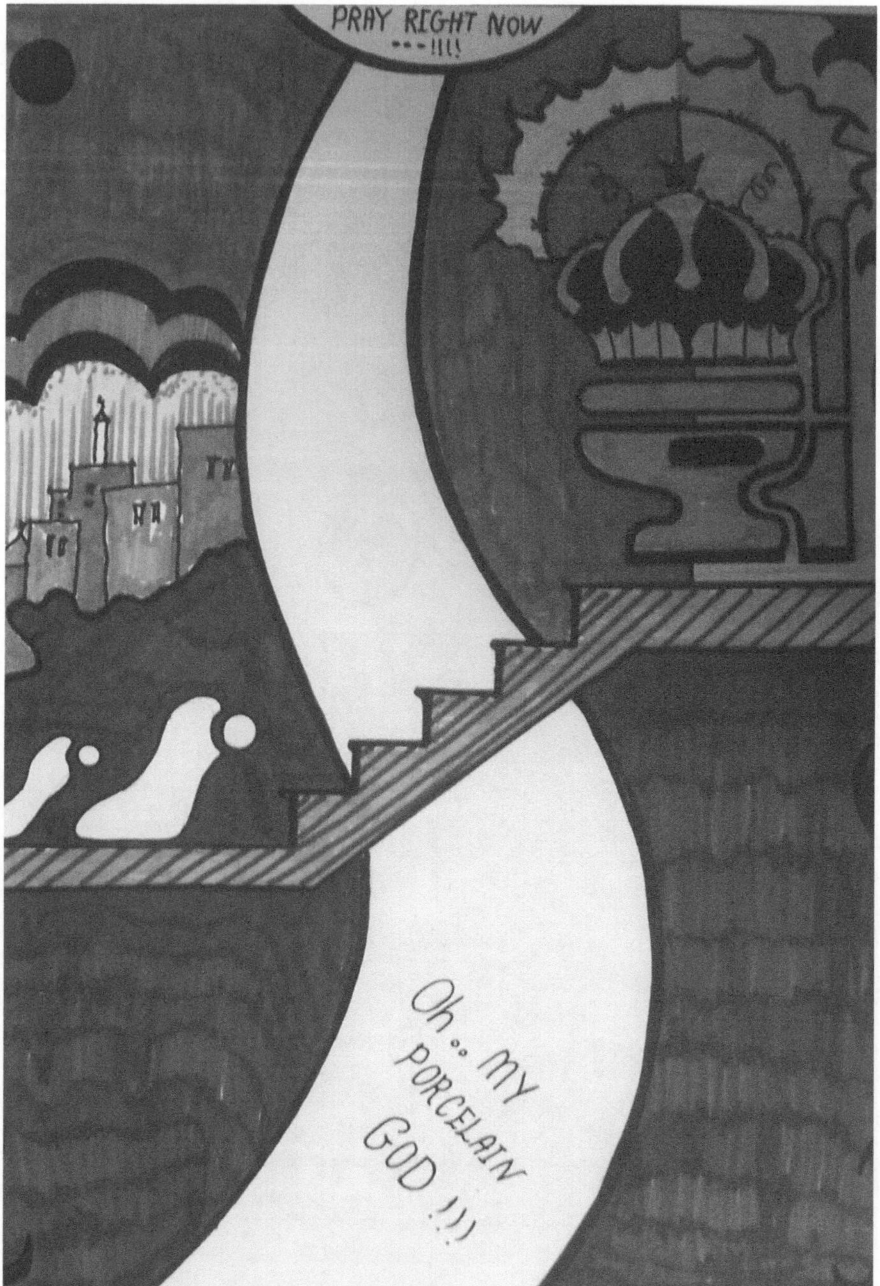

FIGURE 14.2 Miss MS has placed a toilet bowl on an altar and captioned the drawing "Oh . . . My porcelain GOD". She likens the act of self-induced vomiting to the ritual of praying to God. This drawing reflects the compelling and overwhelming power of this compulsion and illustrates the ritual nature of self-induced vomiting which characterizes eating disorders.

Unfortunately, this improvement did not last for more than one year. The relapse was precipitated by the stress of the poor relationship with her family and the break-up of a romantic relationship with a boyfriend. During the course of her illness, she was able to express her feelings and emotions in paintings, which reflected the damaging effect of anorexia nervosa on her life and personality.

Natural course and outcome

Most follow-up studies have been carried out in the West. Short-term follow-up studies suggest that anorexia nervosa runs a fluctuating course with exacerbations and periods of partial remission. Outcomes of the condition are variable; although weight and menstrual functioning usually improve, eating habits often remain abnormal and some patients develop bulimia nervosa. Longer-term studies show that the disorder may run a chronic course and reported mortality rates from long-term follow-up studies of severe cases are high, at around 20%.[18] About 20% of patients make a full recovery and the same proportion remain severely ill; the remainder show some degree of continuing psychiatric disturbance.[19] At least two factors appear to predict outcome. These are: late age at onset (18 years or older) or those with a long history of disease. Individuals with these characteristics tend to fare less well. Some studies suggest that after many years of illness, recovery may take place although it is uncommon.[19,20]

Since most studies have focused primarily on patients with anorexia nervosa, not as much data is available on patients who meet criteria for bulimia nervosa alone. Some community-based studies of bulimia nervosa have suggested that many cases are transitory and tend to resolve over time. One study reported that among patients suffering from bulimia nervosa, the number who met the full criteria for the disorder decreased as time went on. However, 30% continued to engage in recurrent bingeing and purging at 10-year follow-up.[21] Consistent predictors of outcome are yet to be discovered.

Evidence from the Shuriquie and Abdulhamid study indicates that in Arab countries, eating disorders have a similar chronic course to that described in Western reports.[17] However, the sample size in this study is too small to make concrete conclusions.

MET appears to be effective in patients who were motivated to change and who are able to follow up on regular basis. Fluoxetine appears to be mildly effective in reducing episodes of binge eating. Good prognostic features include being motivated to engage in a long-term therapeutic relationship, being employed, and having a family who understands the nature of the illness and provides the patient with support and supervision. Bad prognostic features include: having frequent episodes of binge eating, psychiatric co-morbidity, and having a hostile, over-involved, unsupportive family who has a poor understanding of the nature of the illness. Marriage does not appear to be protective.

Detection

Given that one of the poor prognostic factors in patients with eating disorders is a history of long duration of the disorder, it is likely that early detection and treatment may improve outcome. Therefore, the primary care provider should be aware of individuals among their patients, particularly adolescents, who may suffer from abnormal eating attitudes and monitor their progress.

In the primary care setting, a number of questions might be useful to screen for disordered attitudes toward eating. These include:

- Are you satisfied with your eating patterns?
- Do you believe that you are fat although others say that you are too thin?
- Does your weight affect the way you feel about yourself?
- Do you feel that food dominates your life?[22]

Currently there is little information from Arab countries about the ways that eating disorders present in primary care settings. However, clinical experience suggests that many patients present to general medical settings with conditions such as: chronic nausea and vomiting, abdominal pain or constipation, unexplained weight loss, frequent orthopedic injuries and overuse syndromes due to excessive exercise, unexplained amenorrhea or infertility, and other psychiatric disorders such as depression and anxiety.

Treatment

The treatment of eating disorders in Arab culture is similar in principle to treatment of eating disorders in Western cultures. Medications are non-specific and do not appear to be very useful. Treatment of eating disorders is mainly psychological, with individual and family work. The individual work includes cognitive therapy, most prominently MET. MET emphasizes the discrepancy between present behavior and broader goals and between self-concept and behavior. The interviewer expresses empathy and acceptance through selective reflective listening. This kind of cognitive behavioral therapy promotes self-efficacy, hope, optimism and self-esteem.

Engaging the family is essential in managing patients. Adopting a non-blaming attitude and using family members as co-therapists are also crucial. The less severe cases presenting with a body mass index above 15 can be treated as outpatients using MET and family therapy, especially if the patient is younger. Older patients are usually treated with MET. More severe cases with a body mass index of less than 15 require admission to a psychiatric unit because of the risk of death. The aim of treatment is the restoration of body weight and the establishment of normal eating habits.

Conclusion

The concept that eating disorders are a Western culture-bound syndrome is not valid any longer. Studies from the Arab world indicate that eating disorders exist within this culture, have a similar prevalence and run a similar natural course to those in Western cultures. However, eating disorders appear to be poorly recognized and under-diagnosed in the Arab world. Therefore it is important to increase people's awareness about the eating disorders through the media. Screening for the presence of abnormal eating attitudes and preoccupation with weight and shape among secondary schools could also be beneficial. Training of doctors and health personnel to establish early recognition and subsequent proper management is essential.

References

1 Lee S, Chiu HF, Chen CN. Anorexia nervosa in Hong Kong: why not more in Chinese? *Br J Psychiatry* 1989; **154**: 683–8.
2 Furnham A, Alibhai N. Cross-cultural differences in the perception of female body shapes. *Psychol Med* 1983; **13 (4)**: 829–37.
3 Nasser M. Eating disorders: the cultural dimension. *Soc Psychiatry Psychiatr Epidemiol* 1988; **23 (3)**: 184–7.
4 Shuriquie N. Eating disorders: a transcultural perspective. *East Mediterr Health J* 1999; **5 (2)**: 354–60.
5 Al-Adawi S, Dorvlo AS, Burke DT *et al.* Presence and severity of anorexia and bulimia among male and female Omani and non-Omani adolescents. *J Am Acad Child Adolesc Psychiatry* 2002; **41 (9)**: 1124–30.
6 Al-Subaie A, al-Shammari S, Bamgboye E *et al.* Validity of the Arabic version of the Eating Attitude Test. *Int J Eat Disord* 1996; **20 (3)**: 321–4.
7 Eapen V, Mabrouk AA, Bin-Othman S. Disordered eating attitudes and symptomatology among adolescent girls in the United Arab Emirates. *Eat Behav* 2006; **7 (1)**: 53–60.
8 Nasser M. Screening for abnormal eating attitudes in a population of Egyptian secondary school girls. *Soc Psychiatry Psychiatr Epidemiol* 1994; **29 (1)**: 25–30.
9 Shuriquie N, Elias T, Abdulhamid M. A study of abnormal eating attitude among Jordanian female college students. *Bahrain Medical Bulletin* 1999; **21 (3)**: 88–90.
10 Bener A, Tewfik I. Prevalence of overweight, obesity, and associated psychological problems in Qatari's female population. *Obes Rev* 2006; **7 (2)**: 139–45.
11 Musaiger AO, Shahbeek NE, Al-Mannai M. The role of social factors and weight status in ideal body-shape preferences as perceived by Arab women. *J Biosoc Sci* 2004; **36 (6)**: 699–707.
12 American Psychiatric Association. Task Force on DSM-IV. *Diagnostic and Statistical Manual of Mental Disorders*: DSM-IV. 4th ed. Washington, DC: American Psychiatric Association; 1994.
13 World Health Organization. *The ICD-10 Classification of Mental and Behavioural Disorders: clinical descriptions and diagnostic guidelines.* Geneva: World Health Organization; 1992.

14 Garner DM, Garfinkel PE. The Eating Attitudes Test: an index of the symptoms of anorexia nervosa. *Psychol Med* 1979; **9 (2):** 273–9.

15 Nasser M. The validity of the Eating Attitude Test in a non-Western population. *Acta Psychiatr Scand* 1986; **73 (1):** 109–10.

16 Button EJ, Whitehouse A. Subclinical anorexia nervosa. *Psychol Med* 1981; **11 (3):** 509–16.

17 Shuriquie N, Abdulhamid M. Eating disorders among Jordanian women: a collective case study. *Arab Journal of Psychiatry* 2005; **16 (1):** 52–61.

18 Theander S. Outcome and prognosis in anorexia nervosa and bulimia: some results of previous investigations, compared with those of a Swedish long-term study. *J Psychiatr Res* 1985; **19 (2–3):** 493–508.

19 Fairburn C. Eating disorders. In: Kendall R, Zeally E, editors. *Companion to Psychiatric Studies.* 5th ed. London: Churchill Livingston; 1993. pp. 525–41.

20 Ratnasuriya RH, Eisler I, Szmukler GI *et al.* Anorexia nervosa: outcome and prognostic factors after 20 years. *Br J Psychiatry* 1991; **158:** 495–502.

21 Keel PK, Mitchell JE, Miller KB *et al.* Long-term outcome of bulimia nervosa. *Arch Gen Psychiatry* 1999; **56 (1):** 63–9.

22 Morgan JF, Reid F, Lacey JH. The SCOFF questionnaire: assessment of a new screening tool for eating disorders. *BMJ* 1999; **319 (7223):** 1467–8.

CHAPTER 15

Substance abuse

(★ *Laeth S Nasir*

Introduction

The use of psychoactive substances by humans is a nearly universal phenomenon, particularly if the use of tobacco and caffeine are considered. The use of some substances can have severe physical, psychological and social consequences for individuals, their families and communities. The sociocultural environment is a major factor that determines whether or not people encounter problems, and what types of problems they might encounter in relation to their use of psychoactive substances.

Definitions

Very little systematic research about substance abuse has been done internationally. The application of definitions and diagnostic criteria created in Western countries may be problematic when applied internationally. The following definitions, while they do not necessarily correspond to those in the international classification systems of the *Diagnostic and Statistical Manual of Mental Disorders*, 4th edition (DSM-IV), and *International Classification of Diseases*, version 10 (ICD-10), may be useful in conceptualizing some of the problems related to substance abuse as they relate to people in Arab countries.

➼ *substance abuse or misuse:* the use of a substance in a way that is not medically, socially or legally sanctioned and/or results in harm to oneself or others
➼ *addiction:* a pattern of substance use that is characterized by recurrent use of a psychoactive drug or drugs, and continued compulsive use despite negative health and/or social consequences

➻ *dependence:* a state of physical adaptation that results in a withdrawal syndrome resulting from rapid discontinuation of a substance. Dependence is not the same as addiction. Dependence may occur with the use of medications such as beta blockers, serotonin re-uptake inhibitors, or even narcotics being utilized appropriately for chronically painful conditions.

➻ *tolerance:* the need for increasing doses of a drug to achieve intoxication or the desired effects. Tolerance to different effects of a substance can occur at variable rates. For example, narcotics produce a number of effects with administration, including euphoria and respiratory depression. With repeated administration, the dose of narcotic required to produce euphoria increases, while the dose causing respiratory depression remains relatively unchanged. Therefore, increasing doses of narcotic will be required to provide the desired euphoric effect, but will progressively increase the danger of respiratory failure.

➻ *relapse:* a return to abusing a substance or substances after a period of abstaining from such use.

TABLE 15.1 Psychoactive substances that are commonly (ab)used

Central nervous system depressants
- alcohol
- sedatives, such as benzodiazepines
- inhalants, such as glue, paint and aerosols
- narcotics, such as heroin

Central nervous system stimulants
- nicotine
- caffeine
- cocaine
- qat (khat)
- amphetamines
- pharmaceutical drugs, such as fenetylline (Captagon)

Hallucinogens
- cannabinoids, such as hashish

Etiology

Substance abuse is best conceptualized as a disease that results from a complex interplay between biological, psychological and social factors. The magnitude and extent of the involvement of individual factors varies from one person to another. The final common outcome of this interaction is often manifested by loss of control over the use of a substance or substances. This use continues despite harm in the physical, social or occupational spheres of the individual's life.

Substance abuse and addiction are seen in all parts of the world, among members of all religions, and in people of every age and both sexes. In Western populations, the lifetime incidence of substance abuse has been estimated to be in the range of 10–20%.

Globally, alcohol is the most common substance abused. The use of illicit drugs is also a common and growing problem, particularly among youth. It is clear that in most Arab countries the prevalence of substance abuse is still quite low compared to other parts of the world. However, studies and reports clearly indicate that rates are rising.

Social and cultural norms significantly affect the definitions and patterns of what constitutes "substance abuse" in a given community. For example, the ritual use of alcohol or other drugs is an important part of religious and other ceremonies in many communities. Also, alcohol may be an integral part of normal group behavior in some settings. In these cases, what constitutes "appropriate use" of alcohol is strongly tied to relevant cultural norms, which may vary greatly across communities. In the case of alcohol use, this blurs the border between what is considered "normal" alcohol intake and "alcohol abuse". To deal with this, some authorities have created a separate category of "problem", "at risk" or "harmful" drinking. These categories are primarily based on epidemiologic studies that show associations between increasing alcohol intake and health problems in defined populations. Therefore, these definitions and categories may not be applicable in all cultures.

International studies suggest that substance abuse is more common among people with lower educational attainment, those who suffer from a psychiatric disorder, and those with a history of previous substance abuse. High rates of co-morbid psychiatric illness and substance abuse have been reported in a study of general psychiatric admissions in Lebanon,[1] and another that evaluated outpatients with schizophrenia in Egypt.[2]

The role of the family

Worldwide, men are three times more likely to suffer from substance abuse problems than are women. The reasons for this are unclear, but it has been hypothesized that cultural pressures cause women to express mental health problems preferentially as "internalized" disorders such as depression and anxiety, while men tend to "externalize" their symptoms as violence and substance abuse. In this paradigm, substance abuse may be seen as an attempt to deal with unresolved conflicts, release tension, or to allow the expression of feelings that would otherwise be unacceptable. Indeed, some behavioral theorists conceptualize substance abuse as a conditioned response that is reinforced by subtle cues within the family. A frequently observed pattern is the family member who uses substances as a way to demonstrate autonomy or as a form of rebellion. The behavior of family members may also inadvertently facilitate or enable drinking or substance abuse, for example by concealing adverse consequences, such as missing work.

Particularly in conservative Muslim families, even one episode of alcohol or other substance use can be a powerful expression of anger and resentment. In some families and communities, such use may be considered the equivalent of self-harm behavior, and will be presented to the healthcare provider for assistance. This scenario should never be ignored or underestimated by the clinician, even if the individual who is the focus of attention denies having a problem. Careful and comprehensive assessment of the situation and family is often warranted in these cases.

Treatment of substance-related disorders should always involve family members; guilt, anger and blame often persist even after sobriety is attained. These unresolved conflicts or family patterns may lead to relapse,[3] or find expression in the development of substance-related disorders by another family member.[4]

Social and cultural factors

Availability and community acceptance of substances of abuse have both been established as major risk factors for substance abuse. As a rule, alcohol and other addictive substances are not readily available in Muslim communities, and their use is more stigmatized than in many other areas of the world. This is likely to contribute heavily to the generally low rates of substance abuse in the region. On the other hand, the correspondingly strong stigma surrounding these substances in the community may serve as a powerful deterrent to patients who wish to seek treatment.

A few studies have explored correlations between religious affiliation and the use of substances. One study from northern Israel reported that among adolescents who reported consumption of alcohol, Jews were more likely to purchase it at pubs, Muslims were more likely to obtain it from friends of the same age, and Christians were more likely to get it from their parents.[5] These findings may reflect the relative sociopolitical positions of these groups. Jews, as the politically dominant group, might feel more free to use alcohol in public to facilitate socializing behavior; Christians would be more likely to use it in a religious setting or in family gatherings; and Muslims might tend to use it covertly in a peer setting. An article that reviewed the results of four studies suggested that problem drinking is more prevalent among Christian youth compared to Muslims who drink alcohol in Israel.[6] However, a survey of university students in Lebanon reported that, although Muslims as a group were much less likely to have ever used alcohol than Christians, among those who had ever used alcohol, there were no significant differences in reported rates of alcohol abuse or dependence between the two groups.[7] Some studies suggest that among Muslims living in countries where alcohol is freely available, there is a tendency for increasing rates of alcohol consumption over time.[8,9]

A number of studies have confirmed the importance of religious beliefs and practice in seeking treatment and preventing relapse. This has been most clearly documented among Muslims in settings where religious practice is a prominent part of the prevailing culture.[10]

Substance abuse in Arab countries

Although few large-scale studies of substance use exist, there have been some indications from the medical literature that even in highly conservative societies, the use of alcohol and other drugs may be more prevalent than previously thought. One study from Kuwait found that 10% of 1048 patients seen in an emergency department had measurable levels of alcohol in their blood.[11] In the United Arab Emirates (UAE), a community-based survey suggested a prevalence rate of substance use or abuse among men of approximately 9%,[12] and approximately 5% of a sample of adolescents in a primary care setting in the UAE admitted to substance misuse.[13] One study from Saudi Arabia reported that more than 5% of a sample of school students inhaled volatile substances such as glue.[14] A number of reports have documented increasing needs for substance abuse treatment centers in Saudi Arabia.[15]

Regional differences in use patterns have been observed; a study that compared substance misusers from two Gulf countries having similar geographic, cultural and ethnic features reported demographic differences among users, and differences in the types of drugs abused.[16] Exposure to other cultures through the media, increased travel, and increasing availability of alcohol and drugs, are thought to be contributing to the growth of substance abuse in the region.

Studies from the Arab world report that the typical substance abuser is a young, unmarried unemployed male with friends who are also users, and often a criminal record.[10,17–21] Several studies report an increased incidence of personality disorders, such as borderline and antisocial personalities, among those who misuse drugs and alcohol, particularly polysubstance abusers.[1,20,22]

Caution in interpreting these results is warranted, however, as the more affluent and well-connected might avoid being detected by these reports. Instead, treatment may be sought privately or abroad to avoid the severe stigma that the individual and family may incur from a diagnosis of substance abuse.[23]

Initiation of substance abuse

It is not unusual for substance users to report exposure to substances of abuse relatively early in life. Among a sample of 350 Palestinian drug abusers, 19% reported that they had begun to use substances at age 15 or younger, and an additional 49% of the sample had begun use between 16 and 20 years of age.[24] A national survey of 3345 Omani secondary school adolescents revealed that about 4% of the sample reported alcohol use, and 4% drug use.[25] A nationally representative sample of high school students in Egypt suggested that some had begun experimenting with drugs or alcohol as early as 12 years of age.[26] A study of drug addicts admitted to hospital in Egypt revealed that nearly 40% had begun to use drugs between 15 and 20 years of age.[27] A similar study of addicts admitted to hospital in Lebanon reported first substance use as young as 13.[28] Sixty-four percent of a sample of individuals in a Saudi treatment center reported initiation of drug or alcohol use before 25 years of age;[29] another study of 423 people in addiction treatment facilities in Saudi Arabia reported that approximately 10% had begun use between 10 and 14 years of age.[10] A study of 40 Bahraini heroin users reported initiation of drug use as early as 12 years of age.[30] The users in these studies and others frequently cited peer pressure, boredom or family problems as the instigating factor for initiation of substance use.[21,31]

TABLE 15.2 Selected factors predisposing to substance abuse

■ male sex
■ family problems
■ psychiatric problems
■ personality disorders
■ family or personal history of substance abuse.

Consequences of substance abuse

The consequences of substance misuse accumulate over time. Therefore, many patients will first present to the health provider with substance-related problems a number of years after the problem begins. This time lapse between initiation of use and presentation often complicates diagnosis and treatment efforts, as the patient has often exhausted the goodwill of family and friends. In addition, medical problems, such as hepatitis B, C or human immuno-deficiency virus (HIV) from intravenous drug use,[32–4] or liver cirrhosis due to alcoholism, may be present. Legal problems, unemployment, neglect, abuse and divorce are only a few of the adverse consequences commonly encountered.

Another major consequence of substance abuse is the stigma that affects the patient as well as his or her family and friends. This stigma may be related to the perception that a substance abuser is harmful to others,[35] and can have consequences for all areas of an individual's life, including social contacts and status, employment and self-esteem. This is particularly true in Arab countries, where family and individual reputation are very important. Although one study from Kuwait suggested relatively lenient public attitudes towards substance abusers,[36] another study suggested that in a number of Arab countries, "drug addiction" was among the most stigmatizing of 18 medical or social conditions listed; the list included items such as "being HIV positive", "being dirty and unkempt" and "having a criminal record for burglary".[37] Other studies emphasize the prevalence of punitive attitudes towards those who abuse substances.[38, 39]

Tobacco abuse

Introduction

Although there is quite an extensive literature regarding the use of tobacco in the Arab world, this section will focus on those aspects of tobacco use that are likely to be useful to the health provider from a clinical standpoint.

The use of tobacco and its widespread use in society illustrate many of the issues that make defining the abuse of a substance a difficult and sometimes ambiguous task. Although tobacco is a well-established cause of disease and premature death, has no accepted medical use, and often results in addiction, it is almost universally tolerated as a recreational drug. Rates of tobacco use in the Arab world are generally accepted to be quite high, particularly among males.[40] The effects of ethnicity, culture and changing societal trends can be seen in the different ways and settings in which people choose to use tobacco: chewed, in snuff, cigarettes, pipes or waterpipes ("argile").[41–3]

Studies from Western countries suggest that the typical pattern leading to the initiation of tobacco use can be conceptualized as a four-stage process beginning with a period of *susceptibility* that occurs during adolescence. During this phase, some adolescents are more susceptible than others to experimentation with tobacco. Factors that lead to individual susceptibility are unclear, but may include exposure to the use of tobacco by role models such as family members. At this point, some individuals will move into the second stage, *early experimentation*, where tobacco is tried at least once. It is during this stage that peer norms and behaviors become more important. Further reinforcement and opportunities for use typically lead to more *regular but intermittent* smoking, and finally, a stable daily habit. *Addiction* is frequently established at this point.[44]

Demographics of tobacco use

Studies from Arab countries generally agree that the age of onset of tobacco use tends to occur in adolescence among males in particular.[45–8] Initiation of tobacco use at younger ages tends to occur in families where others (e.g. father, siblings) also smoke.[42,49–51] Exposure and receptivity to Western media were reported to be risk factors for tobacco use among Egyptian adolescents.[52,53] Several studies suggest that in some countries, high rates of smoking among schoolteachers serve to model tobacco use to students.[48,54] The literature also suggests that young people experience increased rates of smoking upon induction into military service, and admission to university.[55] Another observation made by several studies is that rates of tobacco use tend to increase with increasing age; in contrast, data from the United States suggest that smoking rates peak in the mid-20s and subsequently fall with increasing age.[56]

Studies also suggest that particularly among females, initiation of tobacco use may take place at older ages.[55] This phenomenon likely reflects societal pressures and expectations that apply to women, particularly those who are unmarried. It may also partially reflect concealment; one study from Syria reported that proxy reports obtained from relatives suggested that women's actual tobacco use was twice as frequent as had been suggested in previous research.[57] Discrepancies in self-reported rates were also reported from another study carried out in Israel.[58] Despite this caveat, virtually all studies from the Arab world indicate that girls and women start smoking at older ages, and smoke less than their male counterparts. This assumption is bolstered by studies demonstrating much higher rates of tobacco-related mortality among men in Arab countries.[59] Some studies suggest that higher levels of education and non-traditional lifestyles are linked to increased rates of female smoking.[55,60]

Women's initiation of tobacco use at later ages may also be a manifestation of the phenomenon of substance use as an externalization of inner feelings; several reports indicate high rates of tobacco use among women who are divorced, widowed or who otherwise report high levels of mental distress.[61-3]

Interestingly, one study from Yemen reported that girls in that country tended to initiate cigarette use earlier than boys;[64] although rates of female smoking were lower than those of males in Yemen overall, they are reported to be the highest women's rates in the Arab world.[40] The implications of these findings are unclear, but suggest that significant differences in societal practices and norms with respect to tobacco use exist in the region.

Importantly, studies have shown that among those who have quit, or who wish to quit, both religious and health considerations are important.[55,62,63,65-7] Barriers to quitting have been reported to include lack of knowledge about how to quit[62] and difficulty in refusing offers of cigarettes from friends and acquaintances.[68] The first barrier is easily remediable through education; the second may be more challenging. Rituals surrounding hospitality and courtesy are highly valued in Arab society. Offers of a cigarette or other refreshment serve to put the recipient, the giver and the larger group at ease; therefore, appropriate refusal skills and techniques may need to be developed to help individuals to resist tobacco initiation and relapse.

An approach to smoking cessation

Little work on the implementation of smoking cessation programs has been carried out in the region.[65] However, given the high rates of tobacco use in Arab countries, and the degree of health risk that they represent, it is important for health providers to have a framework for addressing tobacco use and cessation with patients in clinical practice.

The dynamics of smoking cessation resemble the dynamics encountered among those who use any addictive substance. At any given time in a population of smokers, there is a proportion of individuals who wish to quit, and there are also those who are not interested in quitting. Depending on factors such as illness, exposure to educational messages or stress, individuals may move from one readiness state to another. A model of human behavior change (the so-called "transtheoretical" model) has been developed that helps conceptualize the process of behavior change and provides practical guidance to health providers in helping patients to break bad habits.[69]

In this model, behavior change is seen as a continuum of attitudes and behaviors that relate to a person's readiness to change; these are marked by stages. Individuals typically progress through these stages at varying rates, and may move back and forth through the stages a number of times before either the desired outcome is reached or they lose motivation to continue. Understanding where a person's current attitudes and behaviors lie on this continuum is important in order to tailor interventions to the individual's case.

Stages of behavioral change

The first of the stages has been labeled *precontemplation* and is one in which the individual has no interest in or desire to change the behavior in question (e.g. a smoker who is not interested in quitting). Patients who are in this stage are typically detected through screening, as they do not see their behavior as a problem. The next stage, *contemplation*, describes the patient who is thinking about quitting some time in the future. Typically, these patients are ambivalent, and vacillate between wanting to proceed with quitting, and the comfort of the status quo. *Preparation or determination* describes an individual who is on the verge of making a quit attempt, and has begun to take some active steps toward quitting. These patients have spent some time thinking about the problem, and now they are ready to do something. This stage may not last without outside support and a definite plan of action. A patient in the *action* stage is actively involved (and currently abstinent). The patient is considered to be in the *maintenance* stage if he or she has been abstinent for at least six months. During this time, behavior changes typically become consolidated and more secure. *Relapse* is a stage that was not initially included as part of the continuum. However, it has been recognized that lapses, slips and returns to previous habits are probably the norm rather than the exception among the majority of those attempting behavior change.

Tailored interventions for smoking cessation based on the patient's stage of readiness to change

- ⚬ *precontemplation:* if a patient is in precontemplation, further attempts to get them to quit are likely to be futile. Instead, provision of traditional patient education, including a firm recommendation to quit which connects the patient's present clinical situation to his or her smoking status (e.g. "smoking is the cause of your recurrent bronchitis"), if possible, is recommended at this stage. The clinician should follow up at every subsequent visit to detect any movement away from this stage.
- ⚬ *contemplation:* the clinician should display empathy with the patient's predicament, express understanding with the feelings of ambivalence, and support their ability and willingness to consider change. Providing examples and stories of patients who have quit, emphasizing the health benefits of quitting, and the effects on loved ones, are likely to be effective. Although the patient is considering cessation, it is important for the clinician to avoid extended argument with the patient. It is not uncommon for patients to continue their ambivalence for some time before deciding on further progress.
- ⚬ *determination:* at this stage, the patient has decided that change is both necessary and possible. Supporting the patient's decision, and providing a specific

plan for cessation – including setting a "quit date" (a specific day that they plan to quit), planning for problems that might arise, identifying others who might help in the quit attempt, writing any necessary prescriptions and setting a follow-up appointment to review progress – is an effective intervention at this stage.

- *action:* although this stage of behavior change is largely patient-dependent, the clinician can help by providing ongoing support. This might include suggesting ways to deal with withdrawal symptoms, congratulating the patient on his or her progress, and reminding them of the unpleasant aspects of the habit from which they are now free.
- *relapse:* the clinician should help the patient to avoid becoming demoralized, and instead use the lapse as a learning opportunity for future attempts. Excessive expressions of disappointment may shame the patient, discouraging them from making further quit attempts. Rather, discussions of what led to the relapse (e.g. negative emotional states, stress or exposure to high-risk social situations) might be helpful.

Conclusions

As discussed in this chapter, few studies have explored the prevalence or presentations of substance abuse among primary care populations in the Arab world, although the condition is recognized to be increasingly prevalent. Lack of study and discussion in the region is primarily due to the taboo nature of the subject. Even in the healthcare setting, few healthcare professionals feel comfortable asking patients questions that may be perceived to be offensive. Studies exploring the most acceptable way to approach screening in the clinical setting would be a valuable addition to the literature. Another barrier to effective detection and management is the disparity between definitions of what constitutes the "abuse" of a substance. While health professionals tend to apply conventional categories as outlined in the ICD-10 and DSM-IV, Arab families and societies may not distinguish between substance "use", "abuse" and "addiction". This divergence may lead health providers and researchers to fail to recognize that the impact of substance abuse is determined largely by family and community norms and not by the amount or pattern of alcohol or substance use. Recognition of the role of the community in defining the appropriate use of substances, education, early detection, and the development of successful and locally appropriate diagnostic and treatment models, are important steps in the continuing battle against substance abuse. Improvements in public health interventions such as community education about the health effects of tobacco, as well as individual efforts by clinicians and others, will be needed to reduce the impact of tobacco use on society.

References

1 Karam EG, Yabroudi PF, Melhem NM. Comorbidity of substance abuse and other psychiatric disorders in acute general psychiatric admissions: a study from Lebanon. *Compr Psychiatry* 2002; **43 (6):** 463–8.

2 Asaad T, Okasha T, El-Khouly G *et al.* Substance abuse in a sample of Egyptian schizophrenic patients. *Addictive Disorders and Their Treatment* 2003; **2 (4):** 147–50.

3 Al-Nahedh N. Relapse among substance-abuse patients in Riyadh, Saudi Arabia. *East Mediterr Health J* 1999; **5 (2):** 241–6.

4 Demerdash AM, Mizaal H, El Farouki S *et al.* Some behavioural and psychological aspects of alcohol and drug dependence in Kuwait Psychiatric Hospital. *Acta Psychiatr Scand* 1981; **63 (2):** 173–85.

5 Weiss S. How do Israeli adolescents of four religions obtain alcoholic beverages and where? *Journal of Child and Adolescent Substance Abuse* 1995; **4 (4):** 79–87.

6 Weiss S. Review of drinking patterns of rural Arab and Jewish youth in the north of Israel. *Subst Use Misuse* 2002; **37 (5–7):** 663–86.

7 Karam EG, Maalouf WE, Ghandour LA. Alcohol use among university students in Lebanon: prevalence, trends and covariates. The IDRAC University Substance Use Monitoring Study (1991 and 1999). *Drug Alcohol Depend* 2004; **76 (3):** 273–86.

8 Bradby H, Williams R. Is religion or culture the key feature in changes in substance use after leaving school? Young Punjabis and a comparison group in Glasgow. *Ethn Health* 2006; **11 (3):** 307–24.

9 Razvodovsky Y. Influence of culture on attitudes toward alcohol of Arab Muslim university students. *Adicciones* 2004; **16 (1):** 53–62.

10 Qureishi N, Al-Habeeb TA. Sociodemographic parameters and clinical pattern of drug abuse in Al-Qassim region-Saudi Arabia. *Arab Journal of Psychiatry* 2000; **11 (1):** 10–21.

11 Bilal AM, Angelo-Khattar M. Correlates of alcohol-related casualty in Kuwait. *Acta Psychiatr Scand* 1988; **78 (4):** 417–20.

12 Abou-Saleh MT, Ghubash R, Daradkeh TK. Al Ain Community Psychiatric Survey. I. Prevalence and socio-demographic correlates. *Soc Psychiatry Psychiatr Epidemiol* 2001; **36 (1):** 20–8.

13 Abou-Saleh M. Substance use disorders: recent advances in treatment and models of care. *Journal of Psychosomatic Research* 2006; **61:** 305–10.

14 Al-Umran K, Mahgoub O, Quraishi N. Volatile substance abuse among school students of eastern Saudi Arabia. *Annals of Saudi Medicine* 1993; **13 (6):** 520–4.

15 Al-Delaim F. Management of substance abuse in Saudi Arabia. *Derasat Nafseyah* 1997; **7 (3):** 470–84.

16 Taha A. Comparison of patterns of substance abuse in Saudi Arabia and the United Arab Emirates. *Social Behavior and Personality* 2001; **29 (6):** 519–30.

17 Amir T. Personality study of alcohol, heroin, and polydrug abusers in an Arabian Gulf population. *Psychological Reports* 1994; **74:** 515–20.

18 Chaleby K. A comparative study of alcoholics and drug addicts in an Arabian Gulf country. *Soc Psychiatry* 1986; **21 (1):** 49–51.

19 Omer AA, Ezzat BE. Volatile substance abuse: experience from Al Amal Hospital, Jeddah. *Ann Saudi Med* 1999; **19 (4):** 374–5.

20 El-Kshishy H. Personality characteristics correlates in drug abuse. *Derasat Nafseyah* 1996; **6 (4):** 518–57.

21 Suleiman R, Shareef M, Kharabsheh S *et al.* Substance use among university and college students in Jordan. *Arab Journal of Psychiatry* 2003; **14 (2):** 94–105.

22 Amir T. Personality study of alcohol, heroin, and polydrug abusers in an Arabian Gulf population. *Psychol Rep* 1994; **74 (2):** 515–20.

23 Al-Ansari EA, Negrete JC. Screening for alcoholism among alcohol users in a traditional Arab Muslim society. *Acta Psychiatr Scand* 1990; **81 (3):** 284–8.

24 Weiss S, Sawa GH, Abdeen Z *et al.* Substance abuse studies and prevention efforts among Arabs in the 1990s in Israel, Jordan and the Palestinian Authority – a literature review. *Addiction* 1999; **94 (2):** 177–98.

25 Jaffer YA, Afifi M, Al Ajmi F *et al.* Knowledge, attitudes and practices of secondary-school pupils in Oman: I. health-compromising behaviours. *East Mediterr Health J* 2006; **12 (1–2):** 35–49.

26 Soueif MI, Youssuf GS, Taha HS *et al.* Use of psychoactive substances among male secondary school pupils in Egypt: a study on a nationwide representative sample. *Drug Alcohol Depend* 1990; **26 (1):** 63–79.

27 Abou Khatwa SA, Kamel FA, Youssef RM *et al.* Epidemiological study of addicts admitted to Maamoura Psychiatric Hospital in Alexandria. *J Egypt Public Health Assoc* 1997; **72 (1–2):** 87–112.

28 Baddoura C. [Drug addiction in Lebanon.] *Bull Acad Natl Med* 1992; **176 (9):** 1505–14; discussion 1514–15.

29 Iqbal N. Substance dependence: a hospital based survey. *Saudi Med J* 2000; **21 (1):** 51–7.

30 Derbas AN, al-Haddad MK. Factors associated with immediate relapse among Bahraini heroin abusers. *East Mediterr Health J* 2001; **7 (3):** 473–80.

31 Al-Kandari FH, Yacoub K, Omu F. Initiation factors for substance abuse. *J Adv Nurs* 2001; **34 (1):** 78–85.

32 Abalkhail BA. Social status, health status and therapy response in heroin addicts. *East Mediterr Health J* 2001; **7 (3):** 465–72.

33 Watts DM, Constantine NT, Sheba MF *et al.* Prevalence of HIV infection and AIDS in Egypt over four years of surveillance (1986–1990). *J Trop Med Hyg* 1993; **96 (2):** 113–17.

34 Njoh J, Zimmo S. The prevalence of human immunodeficiency virus among drug-dependent patients in Jeddah, Saudi Arabia. *J Subst Abuse Treat* 1997; **14 (5):** 487–8.

35 Coker EM. Selfhood and social distance: toward a cultural understanding of psychiatric stigma in Egypt. *Soc Sci Med* 2005; **61 (5):** 920–30.

36 Bilal AM, Makhawi B, al-Fayez G *et al.* Attitudes of a sector of the Arab-Muslim population in Kuwait towards alcohol and drug misuse: an objective appraisal. *Drug Alcohol Depend* 1990; **26 (1):** 55–62.

37 Room R. Taking account of cultural and societal influences on substance use diagnoses and criteria. *Addiction* 2006; **101 Suppl 1:** 31–9.

38 Qasem FS, Mustafa AA, Kazem NA *et al.* Attitudes of Kuwaiti parents toward physical punishment of children. *Child Abuse Negl* 1998; **22 (12):** 1189–202.

39 Younis YO. Attitudes of Sudanese urban and rural population to mental illness. *J Trop Med Hyg* 1978; **81 (12):** 248–51.

40 Shafey O, Dolwick S, Guindon G, editors. *Tobacco Control Country Profiles* 2003. Atlanta, GA: American Cancer Society; 2003.

41 Ward KD, Eissenberg T, Rastam S *et al.* The tobacco epidemic in Syria. *Tob Control* 2006; **15 Suppl 1:** i, 24–9.

42 Hamadeh RR, Musaiger AO. Lifestyle patterns in smokers and non-smokers in the state of Bahrain. *Nicotine Tob Res* 2000; **2 (1):** 65–9.

43 Idris AM, Ibrahim YE, Warnakulasuriya KA *et al.* Toombak use and cigarette smoking in the Sudan: estimates of prevalence in the Nile state. *Prev Med* 1998; **27 (4):** 597–603.

44 Mayhew KP, Flay BR, Mott JA. Stages in the development of adolescent smoking. *Drug Alcohol Depend* 2000; **59 Suppl 1:** S61–81.

45 Saeed AA, al-Johali EA, al-Shahry AH. Smoking habits of students in secondary health institutes in Riyadh City, Saudi Arabia. *J R Soc Health* 1993; **113 (3):** 132–5.

46 Bener A, al-Ketbi LM. Cigarette smoking habits among high school boys in a developing country. *J R Soc Health* 1999; **119 (3):** 166–9.

47 Gadalla MA, Gabal MS, Khella AK. When and why Ain Shams University students started smoking? *J Egypt Public Health Assoc* 1992; **67 (3–4):** 275–90.

48 Fakhfakh R, Hsairi M, Achour N. Epidemiology and prevention of tobacco use in Tunisia: a review. *Prev Med* 2005; **40 (6):** 652–7.

49 Islam SM, Johnson CA. Influence of known psychosocial smoking risk factors on Egyptian adolescents' cigarette smoking behavior. *Health Promot Int* 2005; **20 (2):** 135–45.

50 Moody PM, Memon A, Sugathan TN *et al.* Factors associated with the initiation of smoking by Kuwaiti males. *J Subst Abuse* 1998; **10 (4):** 375–84.

51 Gadalla S, Aboul-Fotouh A, El-Setouhy M *et al.* Prevalence of smoking among rural secondary school students in Qualyobia governorate. *J Egypt Soc Parasitol* 2003; **33 (3 Suppl):** 1031–50.

52 Islam S. *Correlates of Smoking Behavior Among Egyptian Adolescents.* Alhambra: University of Southern California; 2005.

53 Islam SM, Johnson CA. Western media's influence on Egyptian adolescents' smoking behavior: the mediating role of positive beliefs about smoking. *Nicotine Tob Res* 2007; **9 (1):** 57–64.

54 Maziak W, Mzayek F, al-Moushareff M. Smoking behaviour among schoolteachers in the north of the Syrian Arab Republic. *East Mediterr Health J* 2000; **6 (2–3):** 352–8.

55 Maziak W. Smoking in Syria: profile of a developing Arab country. *Int J Tuberc Lung Dis* 2002; **6 (3):** 183–91.

56 Anon. *Tobacco Use.* Office of Applied Studies; 2001 [cited 2007, 15 May]. Available from: http://www.oas.samhsa.gov/nhsda/2k1State/vol1/ch4.htm

57 Maziak W, Tabbah K. Smoking among adults in Syria: proxy reporting by 13–14-year-olds. *Public Health* 2005; **119 (7):** 578–81.

58 Baron-Epel O, Haviv-Messika A, Green MS *et al.* Ethnic differences in reported smoking behaviors in face-to-face and telephone interviews. *Eur J Epidemiol* 2004; **19 (7):** 679–86.

59 Ezzati M, Lopez AD. Regional, disease specific patterns of smoking-attributable mortality in 2000. *Tob Control* 2004; **13 (4):** 388–95.

60 Bint Ahmad Jaffer Y, Afifi M. Adolescents' attitudes toward gender roles and women's empowerment in Oman. *East Mediterr Health J* 2005; **11 (4):** 805–18.

61 Maziak W, Asfar T, Mzayek F. Socio-demographic determinants of smoking among low-income women in Aleppo, Syria. *Int J Tuberc Lung Dis* 2001; **5 (4):** 307–12.

62 Memon A, Moody PM, Sugathan TN *et al.* Epidemiology of smoking among Kuwaiti adults: prevalence, characteristics, and attitudes. *Bull World Health Organ* 2000; **78 (11):** 1306–15.

63 Radovanovic Z, Shah N, Behbehani J. Prevalence of smoking among currently married Kuwaiti males and females. *Eur J Epidemiol* 1999; **15 (4):** 349–54.

64 Bawazeer AA, Hattab AS, Morales E. First cigarette smoking experience among secondary-school students in Aden, Republic of Yemen. *East Mediterr Health J* 1999; **5 (3):** 440–9.

65 Maziak W, Eissenberg T, Klesges RC *et al.* Adapting smoking cessation interventions for developing countries: a model for the Middle East. *Int J Tuberc Lung Dis* 2004; **8 (4):** 403–13.

66 Maziak W, Ward KD, Mzayek F *et al.* Mapping the health and environmental situation in informal zones in Aleppo, Syria: report from the Aleppo household survey. *Int Arch Occup Environ Health* 2005; **78 (7):** 547–58.

67 Nassar NT, Zurayk HC, Salem PA. Smoking patterns among university students in Lebanon. *J Am Coll Health Assoc* 1980; **28 (5):** 283–5.

68 Nierkens V, Stronks K, van Oel CJ *et al.* Beliefs of Turkish and Moroccan immigrants in The Netherlands about smoking cessation: implications for prevention. *Health Educ Res* 2005; **20 (6):** 622–34.

69 Russell ML. *Behavioral Counseling in Medicine: strategies for modifying at-risk behavior.* New York: Oxford University Press; 1986.

CHAPTER 16

Depression, self-harm behavior and suicide

(★ *Laeth S Nasir*

Introduction

Depression is a normal affective state, and expresses the human need for connection and assistance. Experiencing depression is a normal response that may occur in the face of a significant discrepancy between what is hoped for and actual performance. In the context of day-to-day life, this unpleasant emotion serves as a motivator to improved performance. However, depression becomes pathological when it is persistent, pervasive and interferes with such everyday tasks as interpersonal relationships and occupational functioning. One of the difficulties in recognizing pathological depression is that it often arises insidiously, and so goes unrecognized by both the patient and family.

Major depression is one of the leading causes of morbidity worldwide.[1] Particularly in developing countries, the incidence is rising rapidly. This is thought to be largely due to urbanization, increasing stress, and the loss of traditional agrarian lifestyles.[2] In the Arab world, studies have estimated the prevalence of depression in community samples to range between 12% and 32%.[3] Higher rates have been reported from studies of patients in primary care settings.[4]

Internationally, depression is more prevalent in women than men. However, in some Arab countries, the ratio between men and women might be higher than reported elsewhere.[5] A number of factors may contribute to this. The relatively disadvantaged societal position of women in some populations is likely to be one factor.

Loss of traditional psychosocial support may occur with the transition to an urbanized lifestyle. Expectations of the wife to work, and in addition continue to carry out traditionally mandated duties such as household maintenance and childcare, may create additional pressure. Studies confirm that a large number of children in the home is a risk factor for depression.[3,5]

Women who are in polygamous marriages appear to be at particularly high risk of depression,[6-8] although causality is unclear. Domestic violence is also a major risk factor for depression.[6,9,10] In younger women, intergenerational conflict seems to play a major role in the genesis of depression. When seeking treatment, women may face social obstacles in accessing care. They also tend to be more prone to family monitoring of patient–physician communication.[11] Younger women and their families may fear that the stigma of mental illness will reduce their social worth, and consequently, their marriageability.[8]

A number of other risk factors for mental distress and depression have been proposed in the medical literature from Arab countries, including low socioeconomic status, a large number of children in the home, and lower self-efficacy.[12] Cigarette smoking in adolescents,[13] and being a member of a polygamous family,[14,15] have also been reported to be associated with depression.

TABLE 16.1 Selected risk factors for depression in the literature from Arab countries

- low socioeconomic status
- large number of children in the home
- wife or children in polygamous marriage
- cigarette smoking in adolescents.

Self-harm behaviors and suicide

Although studies have consistently shown a high prevalence of depression and psychosocial distress in the Arab world, the available evidence does not indicate a correspondingly high incidence of suicide. Some authorities point to the central role played by religion in Arab society, and its role in discouraging suicide.[7] Others have hypothesized that, as in other collective societies, psychological distress is expressed through help-seeking behavior, manifesting as somatic symptoms such as paralysis, fainting or seizures. These behaviors trigger social support systems to provide increased psychosocial support and reductions in stress. As a society moves towards an individualist model and away from mechanisms that provide close interpersonal contact and intense social support, psychological distress escalates to self-harm behaviors. These behaviors may include substance abuse and suicide.

Substance abuse, parasuicide (defined as self-harm behaviors that fall short of completed suicide) and suicide do occur, and may be concealed by family and even the authorities because of the associated social stigma[16,17] (*see* Chapter 15, Substance abuse). Social factors may also affect the incidence of self-harm behavior. One study[18] showed that the rates of parasuicide in Jordan were consistently lower during the month of Ramadan than during the months that preceded or followed it. Studies suggest that parasuicide and suicidal behavior in adolescents are frequently related to family disputes or academic failure.[7,16,17,19] Parasucidal behavior is most frequently seen in individuals suffering from an adjustment disorder. There is some evidence that in adolescents, being in a "boyfriend" or "girlfriend" relationship is a risk factor for parasuicidal behavior.[16] Virtually all studies agree that the most common self-harm behavior is self-poisoning with over-the-counter analgesics or prescribed medications. Older patients tend to have a higher suicidal intent than adolescents.[20,21] Reports from Jordan, Palestine, Israel and Egypt indicate that self-immolation is not infrequently seen as a cause of suicide, particularly among women.

TABLE 16.2 Risk factors for self-harm or parasuicide from various studies

- female sex
- younger age
- unemployment
- previous attempts
- non-intact family
- wife in a polygamous marriage
- educational failure
- large family size
- psychiatric disorder.

Presentation of depression

Depression is an illness that strikes up to 25% of people at some time in their lives. There is no test or study that will diagnose depression. Just as disease entities such as myocardial infarction or appendicitis may present in many guises, depression can present in various ways. In addition to a thorough understanding of the many manifestations of depression, clinician persistence and flexibility may be necessary to make the diagnosis.

Some authorities report that depressed patients in Arab countries very frequently present with somatic symptoms. These authors report that agitation, insomnia, somatic fixation, impotence and hypochondriasis tend to be prominent symptoms.[22,23] Certainly, these symptoms are common in depression. However, clinical experience and at least one study from the region demonstrate that the majority of these patients will admit to affective symptoms when asked directly.[24,25]

There may be several reasons for the reported prominence of somatic symptoms. First, many patients may perceive that somatic symptoms are their "ticket" to see the doctor. This presentation is exacerbated by the traditionally biomedical and authoritarian relationship between patient and physician, in which the role of the physician is to make a purely "medical" diagnosis.

In this model, the patient is expected to present a medical symptom. Other patients may have a physical illness with a co-existing (co-morbid) depression. A minority of patients may not have an awareness or vocabulary to express their feelings of sadness. Some individuals may suspect that their illness is primarily psychiatric, but the perception of stigma and wishful thinking lead them to conceal these thoughts. This is likely to be the case in patients with a lower level of education. Often these patients will resort to somatic metaphors such as "fatigue".[26]

Guilt and feelings of inadequacy may be manifested by social avoidance or "excessive shyness".[27] In devout patients, guilt is frequently manifested by hyper-religiosity, manifested by excessive praying or fasting. Similar symptoms may be seen in patients with mania or obsessive compulsive disorder.

Diagnosing depression

Most commonly, in the primary care setting, depression presents with few or no signs that can be observed. The clinician may note slow speech, a lack of expression and spontaneous movements, or poor grooming. Alternatively, patients may present with somatic symptoms; frequently, these are neurological or gastrointestinal in nature. Commonly, the patient complains of symptoms out of proportion to the exam – such as the pain preventing any activity, or keeping the patient awake at night.

Alternatively, the symptoms might be extremely vague, and present as fatigue or tiredness. These symptoms are frequently overlooked in the chronically ill patient who might be expected to have identical symptoms from his or her co-morbid condition. The variability in presentation of depression mandates a high index of suspicion for depression. Studies carried out in the Arab world have consistently shown poor detection and follow-up of patients suffering from psychological distress.[28-30]

TABLE 16.3 Behavioral indications of possible depression in a primary care setting

- numerous/recurrent somatic symptoms
- anxious/depressed affect
- repeated negative statements
- diminished spontaneity
- poor eye contact
- frequently critical of others, angry or irritable
- diminished tolerance to stress
- poor grooming
- slumping posture.

Asking direct questions about the patient's mood and functioning is more effective than asking general questions. For example, asking "How are you doing?" is rarely sufficient to elicit the information you are looking for. Far more effective is asking closed ended questions such as: "Have you been feeling sad lately?" and "Are you having trouble sleeping?"

Often, rephrasing the questions into ones that incorporate local metaphors for depression, such as "too much thinking" or "tiredness", is helpful.

Bear in mind that patients who are chronically ill, particularly those suffering from significant disability, such as those following stroke or with chronic pulmonary disease, have a very high prevalence of depression.

A common mistake made in the primary care diagnosis of depression is to over-emphasize the importance of the requisite number of symptoms of depression, and to under-emphasize the impact that these symptoms are having on the patient's life. Both components are important in making the diagnosis.

According to the text revision of *Diagnostic and Statistical Manual of Mental Disorders* 4th edition (DSM-IV-TR), five of nine symptoms should be present for two weeks or more to make the diagnosis (*see* Table 16.4). However, patients may still meet criteria for minor depression if they have fewer than five symptoms. A significant proportion of individuals suffering from minor depression will progress to major depression on follow-up. Therefore, detection and early psychosocial intervention may be effective in improving the patient's quality of life and interrupting progression.

TABLE 16.4 Symptoms of depression according to the DSM-IV-TR

- depressed mood
- diminished interest or pleasure (anhedonia)
- energy loss or fatigue
- weight or appetite loss or gain
- insomnia or hypersomnia
- psychomotor retardation or agitation
- thoughts of worthlessness or feelings of guilt
- indecisiveness or poor concentration
- thoughts of self-harm or death.

In addition to symptoms, the severity and pervasiveness of the symptoms must be considered. Most importantly, to make a diagnosis of depression it must be clear that symptoms are interfering with the patient's life. They should also be shown to cause a noticeable or significant diminution of function from the premorbid level.

To detect interference with function, it is important to assess the areas of work (or school, for students), interpersonal interactions such as relationships with family and friends, religious activities and recreational activities. Finally, the intrapersonal environment should be evaluated, including feelings of psychic discomfort, poor self-esteem, chronic discouragement or lack of positive feelings about the future.

To assess severity of depression, the clinician should assess how much of an overall burden the depression represents in the patient's life. Asking about the amount of disability that patients experience is one way to do this: "How are you functioning at work (school)?", "Do you enjoy sitting with people as much as you used to?", "Are you having trouble meeting your family obligations?", "Have you lost interest in doing things you used to do?" A patient with many severe and unremitting depressive symptoms would be classified as having a more severe depression than one with few symptoms in a discrete area. Some symptoms, such as catatonia or psychosis, necessarily mark the depression as being severe and usually warrant hospitalization because of potentially dangerous consequences.

An important part of the patient evaluation is the family history. Individuals with a positive family history of depression are at approximately three times higher risk of depression than those without this history. Taking the family history may be one of the most sensitive parts of the interview. Even if patients are willing to accept that they may have a psychiatric condition, they may not be willing to reveal negative information or speculate about other family members. For this reason, the clinician may choose initially to ask about other family members only in regards to their occupations and general levels of functioning. Indirect clues of psychiatric illness might include family members who had previously been employed but are now dependent on family for unclear reasons. If the clinician does directly question about a family history of mental illness, positive responses will be maximized if the question is phrased "Who else in your family suffers from this?" and not "Does anyone else suffer from this?".

Precipitants of depression

Frequently, a precipitating event for the onset of depression cannot be found. However, any stressful situation can trigger depression. These situations can include family disruption, loss of a loved one or of other important relationships, immigration, and academic, occupational or economic stressors. Often, post-traumatic stress disorder is a co-morbid condition in patients who have experienced violence.

Both alcohol and substance abuse can be secondary causes of depression. Alternatively, substance abuse may represent patient attempts to reduce the symptoms of an underlying affective disorder. A number of studies have linked cigarette smoking to mental distress, but the causal relationship is unclear.[13,31]

Asking about suicidal intent

Healthcare professionals often find it difficult to ask about suicide. Some fear that by asking about it, they may plant the idea in the depressed person's mind. Others fear that this question will embarrass patients or frighten them unnecessarily. In practice, the clinician should explore the patient's thoughts of possible self-harm whenever a patient is encountered who seems to be hopeless, or expresses feelings of helplessness. Such exploration might include a comment like: "Sometimes people start to think about their own life and whether it is worth living." This might be followed by: "Have you been thinking about death?", "How often do you think about it?", "Are you afraid of death?" (also frequently elicits feelings of guilt and self reproach).

Some patients will deny suicidal preoccupation, but may reply affirmatively if asked: "Do you wish God would let you die?" A positive response may be explored further by asking: "How do you think that would happen?"

How to ask about suicidal intent
- Ask directly: "Have you thought of harming yourself?"
- If negative, ask: "Do you wish God would let you die?", "How would that happen?"

Making the diagnosis

If a diagnosis of depression is made, the patient may request that accompanying family members not be informed of the true diagnosis. This may create a delicate situation for the clinician. Depending on the situation, the clinician may want to counsel the patient that it might be in his or her best interests for family members to know the diagnosis. The discussion may need to involve family members who are not present. In some families, it may be necessary to reach consensus with decision-makers before beginning a course of treatment, and even before a diagnosis is accepted.

Some individuals may feel that depression is due to a character defect, or faulty child-rearing practices. The fact that depression is an illness like any other and is not the patient's or the family's fault should be specifically addressed with all patients. It is not unusual for patients and families to strongly resist or reject a diagnosis of depression. The turmoil that this can potentially cause can lead to an understandable reluctance on the part of healthcare providers to pursue this diagnosis aggressively.

It is important for the clinician to acknowledge the sensitivity of the subject, and to explore the implications of the diagnosis with the patient, and perhaps family decision-makers. It is also important to assure the patient and family of complete confidentiality. Follow-up discussions should incorporate patient education to maximize patient adherence to long-term treatment of the condition and relapse prevention. Several important points should be stressed:
- immediate results should not be expected
- relapse may occur
- the patient is a central part of the treatment, and is also responsible for progress
- with appropriate management, the patient can live a normal life.

Interventions

Increasing social contacts and social support is a proven and generally non-stigmatizing intervention that can and should be applied to patients suffering from anxiety, minor depression or adjustment disorder. It is also an important adjunctive treatment for patients suffering from major depression. There is no clear evidence that increased social support alone is sufficient to treat major depression. However, a "stepped-care" approach to the treatment of depression may be a reasonable one in certain circumstances if closely monitored by the clinician. A trial of increased social support, patient homework and close observation may lead to resolution or clarification of the situation. It may be useful to hold a meeting with family members to educate, emphasize the importance of their involvement in the course of treatment, and to suggest methods by which this may be accomplished.

Although there is no evidence in the literature from the Arab world regarding preferred treatment modalities for depression, clinical experience suggests that non-pharmaceutical management is often strongly preferred by patients with depression because of popular perceptions that antidepressants are habit-forming or harmful. Counseling with a mental health professional is generally perceived very negatively, as is referral to a psychiatrist.[8,11] Patients are far more likely to be accepting of medical treatment and/or brief counseling if it is delivered by the primary care physician (*see* Chapter 11, Approach to the patient in primary care psychiatry). Some authors report that psychotherapeutic interventions based on traditional Western models are ineffective or counterproductive.[32,33] Physician-directed behavioral interventions are thought to be more successful, but evidence-based literature is lacking. Novel approaches to the delivery of counseling to women suffering from mental distress in developing countries have been described.[8,34] These involve the integration of counseling into traditional social support behaviors.

References

1 Lee S. Socio-cultural and global health perspectives for the development of future psychiatric diagnostic systems. *Psychopathology* 2002; **35 (2–3):** 152–7.
2 Harpham T. Urbanization and mental health in developing countries: a research role for social scientists, public health professionals and social psychiatrists. *Soc Sci Med* 1994; **39 (2):** 233–45.
3 Hamid H, Abu-Hijleh NS, Sharif SL *et al.* A primary care study of the correlates of depressive symptoms among Jordanian women. *Transcult Psychiatry* 2004; **41 (4):** 487–96.
4 Becker S, Al Zaid K, Al Faris E. Screening for somatization and depression in Saudi Arabia: a validation study of the PHQ in primary care. *Int J Psychiatry Med* 2002; **32 (3):** 271–83.
5 Daradkeh TK, Ghubash R, Abou-Saleh MT. Al Ain community survey of psychiatric morbidity II. Sex differences in the prevalence of depressive disorders. *J Affect Disord* 2002; **72 (2):** 167–76.

6 Maziak W, Asfar T, Mzayek F *et al.* Socio-demographic correlates of psychiatric morbidity among low-income women in Aleppo, Syria. *Soc Sci Med* 2002; **54 (9):** 1419–27.

7 Al-Jahdali H, Al-Johani A, Al-Hakawi A *et al.* Pattern and risk factors for intentional drug overdose in Saudi Arabia. *Can J Psychiatry* 2004; **49 (5):** 331–4.

8 Nasir LS, Al-Qutob R. Barriers to the diagnosis and treatment of depression in Jordan: a nationwide qualitative study. *J Am Board Fam Pract* 2005; **18 (2):** 125–31.

9 Maziak W, Asfar T. Physical abuse in low-income women in Aleppo, Syria. *Health Care Women Int* 2003; **24 (4):** 313–26.

10 Roberts GL, Lawrence JM, Williams GM *et al.* The impact of domestic violence on women's mental health. *Aust N Z J Public Health* 1998; **22 (7):** 796–801.

11 Al-Krenawi A. Mental health service utilization among the Arabs in Israel. *Soc Work Health Care* 2002; **35 (1–2):** 577–89.

12 Hamdi N. Relationship of perceived self-efficacy to depression and tension among students of the Faculty of Education, University of Jordan. *Dirasat* 2000; **27 (1):** 44–56.

13 Yunis F, Mattar T, Wilson AK. The association between tobacco smoking and reported psychiatric symptoms in an adolescent population in the United Arab Emirates. *Social Behavior and Personality* 2003; **31 (5):** 461–6.

14 Al-Krenawi A, Graham JR. A comparative study of family functioning, health, and mental health awareness and utilization among female Bedouin-Arabs from recognized and unrecognized villages in the Negev. *Health Care Women Int* 2006; **27 (2):** 182–96.

15 Al-Krenawi A, Graham JR. A comparison of family functioning, life and marital satisfaction, and mental health of women in polygamous and monogamous marriages. *Int J Soc Psychiatry* 2006; **52 (1):** 5–17.

16 Zaidan ZA, Burke DT, Dorvlo AS *et al.* Deliberate self-poisoning in Oman. *Trop Med Int Health* 2002; **7 (6):** 549–56.

17 Daradkeh TK, Al-Zayer N. Parasuicide in an Arab industrial community: the Arabian-American Oil Company experience, Saudi Arabia. *Acta Psychiatr Scand* 1988; **77 (6):** 707–11.

18 Daradkeh TK. Parasuicide during Ramadan in Jordan. *Acta Psychiatr Scand* 1992; **86 (3):** 253–4.

19 Suleiman MA, Nashef AA, Moussa MA *et al.* Psychosocial profile of the parasuicidal patient in Kuwait. *Int J Soc Psychiatry* 1986; **32 (3):** 16–22.

20 Al-Ansari A, Hamadeh R, Matar A *et al.* Overdose among Bahraini adolescents and young adults: psychosocial correlates. *The Arab Journal of Psychiatry* 1997; **8 (2):** 115–24.

21 Hamdi E, Amin Y, Mattar T. Clinical correlates of intent in attempted suicide. *Acta Psychiatr Scand* 1991; **83 (5):** 406–11.

22 Okasha A. Mental health in the Middle East: an Egyptian perspective. *Clin Psychol Rev* 1999; **19 (8):** 917–33.

23 Okasha A. Focus on psychiatry in Egypt. *Br J Psychiatry* 2004; **185:** 266–72.

24 El-Rufaie OE, Al-Sabosy MA, Bener A *et al.* Somatized mental disorder among primary care Arab patients. I. Prevalence and clinical and sociodemographic characteristics. *J Psychosom Res* 1999; **46 (6):** 549–55.

25 El-Rufaie OE, Absood GH. Minor psychiatric morbidity in primary health care: prevalence, nature and severity. *Int J Soc Psychiatry* 1993; **39 (3):** 159–66.

26 McIlvenny S, DeGlume A, Elewa M *et al.* Factors associated with fatigue in a family medicine clinic in the United Arab Emirates. *Fam Pract* 2000; **17 (5):** 408–13.

27 Bassiony MM. Social anxiety disorder and depression in Saudi Arabia. *Depress Anxiety* 2005; **21 (2):** 90–4.

28 Becker SM. Detection of somatization and depression in primary care in Saudi Arabia. *Soc Psychiatry Psychiatr Epidemiol* 2004; **39 (12):** 962–6.

29 Al-Jaddou H, Malkawi A. Prevalence, recognition and management of mental disorders in primary health care in Northern Jordan. *Acta Psychiatr Scand* 1997; **96 (1):** 31–5.

30 El-Rufaie OE. Primary care psychiatry: pertinent Arabian perspectives. *East Mediterr Health J* 2005; **11 (3):** 449–58.

31 Lekka NP, Lee KH, Argyriou AA *et al.* Association of cigarette smoking and depressive symptoms in a forensic population. *Depress Anxiety* 2006; **24 (5):** 325–30.

32 Al-Krenawi A, Graham JR, Ophir M *et al.* Ethnic and gender differences in mental health utilization: the case of Muslim Jordanian and Moroccan Jewish Israeli out-patient psychiatric patients. *Int J Soc Psychiatry* 2001; **47 (3):** 42–54.

33 Al-abdul-Jabbar J, Al-Issa I. Psychotherapy in Islamic society. In: Al-Issa I, editor. *Al Junun: mental illness in the Islamic world.* Madison, CT: International Universities Press Inc.; 2000. p. 382.

34 Ali BS, Rahbar MH, Naeem S *et al.* The effectiveness of counseling on anxiety and depression by minimally trained counselors: a randomized controlled trial. *Am J Psychother* 2003; **57 (3):** 324–36.

PART 4

Patient education

CHAPTER 17

Patient education

(★ *Anahid Kulwicki*

Introduction

Health education is a critical component of patient care, whether it focuses on health promotion, health maintenance or illness prevention. Patients who are in contact with health professionals must be provided with appropriate health information that will arm them with the necessary tools for recovery from health-related conditions and maintenance of healthy lifestyles. With this information, patients can make informed decisions about their health issues, and may be able to tailor recommendations to fit their own lifestyles if needed.

There are many research articles in the Arab world indicating the pressing need for patient educational materials for Arab clients. The first *The Arab Human Development Report* [1] established three cardinal deficits impeding human development in Arab countries: knowledge acquisition, freedom and good governance, and women's empowerment. The deficit in knowledge acquisition has led to the Arab countries falling behind many of the world's developing countries in terms of science, technology and patient education. Making health services accessible to disadvantaged populations, especially in rural areas, tackling the absence of qualified staff and operational equipment, improving literacy, and investing in preventive health, will inevitably improve health conditions and enhance human development in the Arab region.[2] With these advancements, great strides can be made in improving the quality of patient education and healthcare.

In the Arab world, the primary focus of healthcare services continues to emphasize the provision of medical treatment for acute disorders. The medical provider still is considered the primary provider of all medical counseling.

This paradigm is beginning to change with changes in healthcare which include:

⇥ the increasing costs of healthcare
⇥ transitions in population demographics and disease states
⇥ patients becoming more involved in healthcare
⇥ the use of television and other media becoming pervasive.

Patient education is a fairly new topic of discussion in the Arab world, and knowledge about the best methods to impart education is only recently becoming available. A number of Arab countries are currently developing research into patient education – most prominently Libya, the United Arab Emirates (UAE), Saudi Arabia, Jordan, Egypt and Lebanon.

In a study from the UAE examining women's experiences during childbirth, perceptions of patient satisfaction were explored. Using a structured questionnaire, researchers inquired about women's experiences while in the hospital. Results indicated that 13.2% of women had negative experiences, including feelings of anger, fear, sorrow, regret, guilt, jealousy, and even a sense of failure and disappointment.[3] The remainder of the women expressed that their experience was enjoyable, and that they had been well-informed about their perinatal care. It is plausible to suggest that the reason some of the women had such negative experiences was because they had not been adequately educated and prepared for the experience.

Another study from the UAE addressed the issue of how best to educate patients, by examining methods of patient education for patients with diabetes. The study concluded that written and electronic media, as well as contact with a nurse or doctor, were effective sources of education.[4] Reported to be less effective were conversations with significant others, dieticians and pharmacists. This suggests that in order for education to be valuable to the patient, it must come from a medical professional, as well as being in written or electronic forms. This study, however, may have limited applicability to other Arab countries, due to the fact that the UAE has one of the highest rates of Internet use in the world, therefore, the population may have more familiarity and comfort with electronic media in an educational role.

In Libya, one study evaluated the responses to a questionnaire on health knowledge, healthy behaviors, and the impact of various health education media among the general public. The participants of the study ranked health education media by effectiveness, ranking television as the most effective source of education, and booklets and leaflets as the least effective source. The participants felt that television would also be an influential source of information on the practice of healthy behaviors, ranking only behind family influence. Books, magazines, newspapers and school health education were also considered important educational venues to increase health awareness and improve healthy behaviors.[5]

A study conducted to investigate patient satisfaction with primary healthcare services in Saudi Arabia yielded similar results to studies conducted in Libya and the UAE. Of 900 respondents interviewed about their satisfaction with healthcare services, 40% were dissatisfied. Among those who were dissatisfied with healthcare services, 38.9% complained that their health problems and treatments were not satisfactorily explained by their physicians. Twenty-two percent of respondents who were dissatisfied claimed that the physician's explanations were not clear and understandable.[6] These findings imply that other methods of education, for example written information, would have been helpful to these patients.

In Lebanon, the current approach at the American University of Beirut Medical Center (AUBMC) towards patient and family education is a multidisciplinary process that utilizes the principles of "adult learning". The AUBMC has developed a comprehensive educational resource manual that includes both didactic and audiovisual materials on a range of health topics. A multidisciplinary team consisting of physicians, registered nurses, pharmacists, dieticians, and/or physical therapists contributes to patient understanding of disease conditions and ways to improve their health status. The Center utilizes a Multidisciplinary Patient Education Record to document the individualized teaching that is provided to the patient and family. A *Patient and Family Education Manual* has been prepared, following Joint Commission on Accreditation of Healthcare Organization standards of care on utilizing best practices, and in consultation with specialty professionals in the field. The *Patient and Family Education Manual* includes patient leaflets and teaching plans pertaining to all the topics covered. The teaching plan provides a content outline of each leaflet, which gives guidance to the nursing staff on the preparation and actual delivery of patient and family education.

All of the studies conducted in the above Arab nations suggest that there is much room for improvement in the patient education programs currently being used. Aside from the knowledge acquired through talking with medical professionals, patients seem to want education from other sources, primarily from television or written sources. Because the Arab world is unique in its blend of cultures and values, the methods used in the Western world may not be appropriate when applied to Arab nations. In order to evaluate the best methods of patient education, local culture and customs must first be observed and considered.

Cultural issues in patient education: the effect of Arab values

The term "Arabs" refers to inhabitants of the Arab world who speak various dialects of the Arabic language, and who share the beliefs and values of the Arabic culture.[7] Included in the Arab world are 22 countries in the Middle East and North Africa, with a population of over 320 million people.

Health coverage varies among the 22 countries in the Arab world. Many Arab countries do not have national healthcare systems that provide healthcare coverage to their residents. In some countries, health insurance or health coverage may be provided for government employees only, or by private companies. Often, cash payments are expected for patient care services, making it difficult for many to seek medical help. In countries that are economically prosperous, the poor may be covered by national healthcare programs.

Though the majority of Arabs follow the Islamic faith, there are also large numbers of Arab Christians, including communities of Copts, Chaldeans, Assyrians, Maronites, Orthodox Christians and Greek Orthodox Christians. There are also small populations of Jewish heritage.

Family roles

Family and kinship ties are highly valued among Arabs. Members of the extended family are expected to be a part of all aspects of an Arab person's life, including financial matters, marriage, birth, illness and death. The strong need for family support is apparent when an Arab patient is hospitalized. The Arab patient seeks comfort and support from his or her extended family members, and may view visitation limits as a violation of basic rights.[7] Involving both the individual and family in patient education can be helpful in patient recovery.

Arab families express pride in their family members and are protective of their family's reputation. This may lead to family members being secretive about illnesses or health concerns that they perceive to bring shame and embarrassment to the family. Among the illnesses and health problems the family may attempt to conceal are mental illness, mental retardation, genetic or reproductive disorders, and chronic illnesses like cardiac disorders and seizures.[8] Elders hold a prestigious position in Arab families, and are looked up to because of their worldly experience. Children are raised to be obedient and never to question their elders. This respect for elders leads to a sense of duty about their care, which may mean that families will often reject medical advice for specialized care or institutionalization for the elderly.

Gender roles

Many Arabs maintain strictly defined gender role differences, and cultural values related to religion. Sex roles may play an important part in health-seeking behaviors.[9] Traditionally, men are the providers and are in charge of social and political matters, while women are the childbearers and caretakers, in charge of household activities.[10] In the healthcare setting, the man of the family is often responsible for the final decisions, and for signing consent forms and surgical permits.[7] Another source of possible conflict is the tradition of discussing sexual matters only between members of the same gender. Males and females generally do not discuss topics that are sexual in nature with members of the opposite sex, even between spouses.[7] This may result in problems with communicating information of a sexual nature to patients of the opposite gender. Also frequently reserved only for talk between same-sex groups is the childbirth experience. Childbirth is considered a female experience, with men generally excluded from the process.[10]

Literacy rates in Arab nations

Literacy rates in Arab nations are low, especially in rural areas and among women and socio-economically disadvantaged populations. In more economically prosperous countries, literacy rates are higher. Overall, the Arab states have some of the lowest adult literacy rates in the world, with over 60% of the region's population over age 15 unable to read and write in 2000, compared to the world literacy rate of 80%.[11] In the region's lesser developed countries, the literacy rates are even lower. Less than 50% of the adult population is able to read and write in countries like Iraq, Yemen and Morocco.[11] In countries like Jordan, Lebanon and Bahrain, literacy rates are relatively high, and above the world average. The literacy rates are also divided by gender, with women accounting for nearly two-thirds of the illiterate population in Arab nations.[11]

In populations with large numbers of illiterate or poorly literate citizens, developing strong patient education programs can be especially difficult. Providing educational materials that do not involve reading is often challenging. This may mean that patients must spend more time with medical health professionals, receiving verbal explanations, and fewer patients can simply be given literature and sent on their way. Another difficulty is that medical education materials are sometimes written in classical Arabic, utilizing terms or expressions that are not easily understood by the average patient. Therefore, efforts must be made to develop materials that can be easily understood by local populations.[12]

Attitudes toward modern medicine

The Arab culture shows great respect for science and advanced knowledge. Most people are aware of Arab historical contributions to medicine and take pride in them. Doctors and other medical experts are viewed as having a power and authority emanating from their knowledge of science and medicine.[7] At least partly because of this deep respect for medical experts, patients often have difficulty questioning medical authorities and making medical decisions. Often, doctors are expected to make health decisions with little or no consultation. In cases where doctors ask for the patient's input in the decision-making process, patients may lose trust in the medical professional and discontinue treatment.[8]

Developing a culturally appropriate education model

Based on difficulties encountered by Arabs in receiving healthcare services, there is a need for culturally specific health promotion and disease-prevention educational materials to be developed and made available to state and local health agencies.[8] Some important considerations that must be made when developing education materials for Arab populations:

➼ some are illiterate or have only a rudimentary education; comprehensive health education programs need to be developed so that they can be understood by people at that education level. Teaching materials should consist of simple messages with familiar words

- educational materials should be aimed at promoting healthy lifestyle behaviors, such as physical examinations, diet, exercise and stress-reduction
- mass media campaigns for health education should be implemented through television and visual aids, such as electronic media and the Internet. These campaigns can be useful in informing the Arab public about common preventable diseases and conditions.

In the Arab world, there is a need to establish a systematic, comprehensive approach to education that takes into account social, economic, cultural and health concerns. Cultural practices, religious beliefs, socioeconomic status and previous experiences must all be considered when planning for patient education.[13] Healthcare providers and researchers must respect the religious and cultural values of the community in which they are working, and remember to consider the basic values of the community members when developing patient education tools. A basic sociocultural understanding is a requirement for the provision of quality healthcare services and adequate patient education.

Common models used in patient education
The Health Belief Model
The Health Belief Model is perhaps the most frequently used theoretical basis for research on patient education. Built from the early work of Kurt Levin, this model focuses on providing a tool for understanding the patient's perception of his or her disease, and the decision-making process he or she uses in the healthcare setting.[14] Using this model, a better understanding of the patient's motivation for seeking services can be obtained.

According to the Health Belief Model, an individual is likely to seek out healthcare services in the following situations:
- the patient perceives that he or she has a disease or condition, or is likely to contract one
- the patient believes that the disease or condition is harmful and has serious consequences
- the patient trusts that the suggested health intervention is appropriate and of value
- the patient believes that the effectiveness of the treatment is worth the cost and effort.[14]

Demographic variables, such as age, gender, ethnicity and socioeconomic status are known to affect an individual's perception of their disease or condition, and can determine whether the individual will perceive his or her problem to be harmful enough to seek medical attention.[15] Other variables that can affect an individual's decision to seek help include advice from friends and family, mass media campaigns, newspaper and magazine articles, or the illness of a loved one.[14]

Research on the Health Belief Model indicates that the costs and barriers an individual confronts as a result of their disease or condition are the most significant factors determining whether or not a patient will seek healthcare services or engage in preventive health behavior.[16] Other variables, such as perceived vulnerability to illness and perceived illness severity, were not as powerful in predicting healthcare-seeking behavior.

While the Health Belief Model is widely used, it has been criticized for being difficult to test, as it is not quantifiable. Furthermore, a direct link between beliefs and behavior has not been proven by the model or by social psychology as a whole.[16] It has also been stated that the model fails to account for significant variables such as public policy and community factors, and does not give a comprehensive view of the variables involved in a patient's perception of his or her disease.[14]

Self-efficacy

Another theoretical basis for patient education is Self-Efficacy Theory, also referred to as Social Learning Theory. This model accounts for personal characteristics of the learner, as well as providing direction to the teacher for managing the social and physical environment of the learner. According to this model, the self-confidence necessary to perform certain behaviors comes from four discrete sources of information – namely, personal mastery, verbal persuasion, vicarious experiences and physiological feedback.[17]

Of the four sources for self-confidence, *personal mastery* is the most important. This refers to the patient's perceived confidence that he or she is performing the desired behavior. An example of personal mastery is the patient's recovering from major surgery and being able to complete his or her physical therapy exercises successfully. If the patient had experienced great difficulty in accomplishing these exercises, or had been unable to finish them correctly, the sense of personal mastery would be diminished, making learning more difficult.[14]

Verbal persuasion is helpful as a source of information for patients, reinforcing their ability to enact new behaviors related to their healthcare. Verbal persuasion can be anything from simple reassurance from healthcare professionals that the patient is competent in his or her new behaviors, to follow-up phone calls and visits to coach the patient through their recovery or new life changes. This encouragement and guidance is helpful for keeping patients on track and their self-confidence high.

Observing role models, or having *vicarious experiences* through other people, is another important source for patients' self-confidence. Possible role models include other patients, healthcare professionals or family members. For example, if a newly diagnosed diabetic patient has a diabetic mother, the new task of performing home blood glucose monitoring will not be so daunting, because the patient has likely seen his or her mother perform the task many times. In this situation, the mother acts as a role model for successful management of the disease, making the patient more comfortable with the new tasks ahead of him or her, thus rendering patient education more effective.

The last source of information for a patient's self-confidence is derived from *physiological feedback*. This refers to the physical cues received by the patient that the new behavior is either appropriate or inappropriate. If the physical cues indicate that the patient is feeling better due to the treatment, the patient will continue on with the behavior. If, however, the treatment makes the patient feel worse, or the physical cues indicate that the course of action is inappropriate, the patient will seek alternative courses of action.

The use of Self Efficacy Theory as a basis for patient education offers a more comprehensive approach than have other methods, like the Health Belief Model, in the past. It has contributed to the theoretical basis of patient education by identifying instruments that increase motivation and enhance learning. The model has been criticized for being too general and for its lack of methodological refinement; but in terms of developing interventions for practice, it provides a useful paradigm for designing programs.[14]

Stress, coping and social support

Stress, coping mechanisms and the modulating effects of social support are very important concepts that are closely related to patient education, and to patients' ability to consider and implement changes in health behavior and health-seeking.

Stress, coping and social support theories are comprised of a group of theoretical perspectives taken from various social scientists.[14] Stress research was historically given momentum by two physiologists, Cannon[18] and Selye.[19] Selye generated the idea that the response of an individual to a given stimulus is more important than the objective nature of the stimulus provoking the response. Other researchers focus on the source of stressors in the person's life. Both of these perspectives are important in understanding some of the dynamics around patient education.[14]

One approach within this family of theories is the *cognitive appraisal approach*, which asserts that the individual's response to a stimulus is unique, and therefore, the evaluation of the stimulus is influenced by individual factors as well as factors from the stimulus itself.[14] Thus, a patient's appraisal of the environment as exceeding available personal resources results in what is perceived as psychological stress.[20] Cognitive appraisal consists of evaluation of perceived problems, as well as potential solutions to these problems.

Lazarus and his colleagues hypothesize that coping is a continuous, ongoing process, comprised of cognitive and behavioral efforts to manage demands that are judged by the patient as exceeding his or her personal resources.[20] Coping resources may include positive beliefs, health and energy, social skills, problem-solving, social support, and material resources. The healthcare provider can assist the patient in developing problem-focused coping by offering information to enhance problem-solving and mobilizing socially supportive resources. One way that this can be accomplished is by educating the patient's family on how to be supportive during times of stress. Health professionals can also help by referring the patient to a social worker or case manager, who can help to identify material resources.

Another approach to stress is the *sociological* view, which hypothesizes that the sources and mediators of stress are found within the social environment of the individual.[21] Stressors consist of life events that can be either physiologic or psychosocial in origin.[22] Mediators of stress are social resources that help the individual to adjust and adapt to the stressors. Social support is a primary mediator of stress, and can help the patient to adapt and move forward from stress.[14] An example would be a supportive spouse helping a patient to recover and encouraging him or her to keep moving forward. This type of support can be a very important factor in the mediation of the patient's stress, and can help them to be more open to education, facilitating their recovery.

Priority-setting in patient education

Patients often experience financial or social issues as a result of, or concurrently with, their disease or condition. When multiple problems exist simultaneously, it may be difficult to prioritize a patient's needs, increasing the complexity of patient education. Outlining a hierarchy of human needs can help health professionals to rank the priority of the problem areas, allowing them to offer guidance and determine the best place to begin patient education.

Maslow theorizes that needs exist in a hierarchy in which lower-level needs must be met before higher-level needs can be achieved.[23] Consideration of this hierarchy of needs can help healthcare professionals to prioritize needs in patient education. The learning process can be severely hampered when a patient's basic needs are not being met. For example, if a patient is in extreme pain, he or she is unlikely to learn much from an educational intervention about the condition until the pain is under control. Until his or her need to feel no pain is resolved, the patient cannot focus on the other need, which is to learn how to manage their disease or condition. To proceed with the educational process, lower-level needs of the patient must be attended to before the introduction of new knowledge is considered.

Preparing materials for patient education

When evaluating and preparing materials for patient education, it is important to examine the goals and objectives of the educational process and determine whether the instructional materials meet those goals. In order to achieve the educational objectives, the healthcare professional must be certain of the materials':

- *accuracy:* are the facts, diagrams, pictures and other visual representations accurate? Errors in the educational material can lead to confusion, and may hinder the patient's ability to learn. Also, the subject matter should be up-to-date. Outdated information can be just as harmful to the patient's education as incorrect information. It is important that the educational materials stay current.

➥ *content:* the subject matter should be representative of all major difficulty areas experienced by patients with the specific medical problem, and should not include irrelevant content. The content should also be appropriate for the intended audience. For example, educational materials intended for children with medical problems should be written at a level that children can understand, with other materials for their parents or guardians written with a higher level of comprehension in mind.

➥ *educational methods:* the materials should be organized in a way that makes sense to the patient and is relatively easy to follow. Major content areas should be highlighted or emphasized so that patients can put the new knowledge into perspective, and terms and concepts should be presented in an appropriate order. For example, it would be inappropriate to begin with a difficult concept; a better method is to start with simple concepts and then move into more complex subject matter. A summary of the concepts and terms should also be included, so that the patient can have the best possible chance of fully comprehending their problem.

➥ *communication:* it is important that the reading level of the material is appropriate for the stated audience. Whenever possible, statements should be clear and direct, without an abundance of medical jargon that will confuse the reader. Feedback should also be available so that the patient can be assured of his or her mastery of the facts, concepts and principles presented. Another key factor to the patient's understanding is the technical quality of the material. The print size, diagrams, spacing and layout of the materials should be appropriate and simple to read. Lastly, it is important that the material be available for the patient to take home, so that the patient can refresh their memory about the details of their condition whenever necessary.

➥ *cost effectiveness and practicality:* the material should not be excessively costly, or it may make providing it impractical. If the same learning objectives may be reached with a more cost-effective option, practicality dictates that the lower-cost materials be used.[14]

Evaluating learning outcomes of patient education

To be effective educators, healthcare professionals must be able to assess or measure not only knowledge acquisition by the patient, but ultimately the behavioral changes based on the patient education that was provided. There are a variety of approaches in evaluating outcomes of patient education, including return demonstration, questionnaires, pre- and post-testing, interviews and direct observation. These approaches include both short- and long-term evaluation. Short-term evaluation involves observing behavioral changes of patients after reviewing health education materials in order to determine whether the selected educational method improved patient behavior. Long-term evaluation is more complex and involves a comprehensive assessment of the behavior changes, as well as determining whether the health status of the individual has improved over time. Surveys can be useful in determining the overall health status of patients.

In conclusion, patient education is a pressing concern in the Arab world, requiring an understanding of patient needs and characteristics including factors such as educational and economic status as well as cultural and religious background. Selecting an appropriate method of teaching is very important to the success of patient education. In order to ensure a satisfactory outcome, all factors related to a patient's ability to learn about health issues should be taken into consideration, and utilized where feasible. With further advancements in patient education for the Arab world, greater human development can be accomplished, and healthcare will improve as a result.

References

1 United Nations Development Programme. Regional Bureau for Arab States, Arab Fund for Economic and Social Development. *The Arab Human Development Report 2002: creating opportunities for future generations.* New York: United Nations Development Programme, Regional Bureau for Arab States; 2002.

2 Boutayeb A, Serghini M. Health indicators and human development in the Arab region. *Int J Health Geogr* 2006; **5:** 61.

3 Rizk DE, Nasser M, Thomas L *et al.* Women's perceptions and experiences of childbirth in United Arab Emirates. *J Perinat Med* 2001; **29 (4):** 298–307.

4 Abdullah L, Margolis S, Townsend T. Primary health care patients' knowledge about diabetes in the United Arab Emirates. *East Mediterr Health J* 2001; **7 (4–5):** 662–70.

5 Elfituri AA, Elmahaishi MS, MacDonald TH. Role of health education programmes within the Libyan community. *East Mediterr Health J* 1999; **5 (2):** 268–76.

6 Ali M, Mahmoud M. A study of patient satisfaction with primary health care services in Saudi Arabia. *Journal of Community Health* 1993; **18 (1):** 49–54.

7 Kulwicki A. People of Arab heritage. In: Purnell L, Paulanka B, editors. *Transcultural Health Care.* 2nd ed. FA Davis; 2004.

8 Kulwicki A. Health issues among Muslim families. In: Aswad B, Bilge B, editors. *Family and Gender Among Muslims: issues facing Middle Eastern immigrants and their descendants.* Philadephia: Temple University Press; 1996. pp. 187–207.

9 Kulwicki A. An ethnographic study of illness perceptions and practices of Yemeni-Americans. *Journal of Nursing Scholarship* 1987; **26 (1):** 13–17.

10 Kulwicki A. Arab women. In: Julia M, editor. *Constructing Gender: multicultural perspectives in working with women.* Australia: Brooks/Cole; 2000. pp. 89–108.

11 Page JE, UNESCO, Basic Education Division. *The Literacy Decade: getting started, 2003–2004.* Paris: Basic Education Division, Literacy and Non-Formal Education Section; 2004.

12 Nasir L, Nasir A. Introducing Arabic language patient education materials in Jordan. *Patient Education and Counseling* 2006; **60:** 142–5.

13 Jarrah SS, Halabi JO, Bond AE *et al.* Iron deficiency anemia (IDA): perceptions and dietary iron intake among young women and pregnant women in Jordan. *J Transcult Nurs* 2007; **18 (1):** 19–27.

14 Rankin SH, Stallings KD. *Patient Education: issues, principles, practices.* 3rd ed. Philadelphia, PA: Lippincott-Raven Publishers; 1996.

15 Janz NK, Becker MH. The Health Belief Model: a decade later. *Health Educ Q* 1984; **11 (1):** 1–47.

16 Rosenstock I. The Health Belief Model: explaining health behavior through expectancies. In: Glanz K, Rimer BK, Lewis FM, editors. *Health Behavior and Health Education: theory, research, and practice.* 3rd ed. San Francisco: Jossey-Bass; 2002. pp. xxx, 583.

17 Bandura A. *Social Learning Theory.* Englewood Cliffs, NJ: Prentice Hall; 1977.

18 Cannon WB. *The Wisdom of the Body.* New York: WW Norton & Company; 1939.

19 Selye H. *Stress in Health and Disease.* Boston: Butterworths; 1976.

20 Lazarus RS, Folkman S. *Stress, Appraisal, and Coping.* New York: Springer Pub. Co.; 1984.

21 Pearlin LI, Lieberman MA, Menaghan EG *et al.* The stress process. *J Health Soc Behav* 1981; **22 (4):** 337–56.

22 Pearlin LI, Schooler C. The structure of coping. *J Health Soc Behav* 1978; **19 (1):** 2–21.

23 Zalenski RJ, Raspa R. Maslow's hierarchy of needs: a framework for achieving human potential in hospice. *J Palliat Med* 2006; **9 (5):** 1120–7.

Index